Atlas of
Uncommon
Pain
Syndromes

Additional titles from the frontlines of pain management by Steven D. Waldman, M.D., J.D.

Interventional Pain Management, 2nd Edition   ISBN 0-7216-8748-2

This clinically oriented, practical text offers comprehensive how-to guidance on the full spectrum of pain management. Sixty-two leading experts discuss general topics, cost-effective treatments, possible complications, advances in pain control, and the rapid growth and timely changes affecting the specialty. More than 600 illustrations, and 18 all-new chapters, demonstrate the intricacies of the latest procedures—in crisp detail.

Atlas of Interventional Pain Management, 2nd Edition (In Press)

ISBN 0-7216-0108-1

"A nice addition to the pain management physician's library."—Anesthesiology

New edition of this best-selling text features more than **100 new radiographs, CTs, and MRIs**, which provide unparalleled guidance in performing interventional pain procedures. **Twenty new chapters**, including Radiofrequency Lesioning—Sphenopalatine Ganglion; Cervical Epidural Block—Translaminar Approach; Genitofemoral Nerve Block; Percutaneous Vertebroplasty; and much more! A reader-friendly "how-to-do-it" approach demonstrates common interventional pain management techniques. Step-by-step full-color illustrations and concise bulleted text explore procedures for all major anatomic sites. For each procedure you'll also find potential pitfalls, clinical pearls, and CPT-2002 coding.

Atlas of Pain Management Injection Techniques   ISBN 0-7216-8504-8

"A quick reference source on a variety of peripheral injection techniques."—Mayo Clinic Proceedings

Here's outstanding guidance on performing a complete range of clinical injection procedures—from the head and neck to the ankle and foot! Concise step-by-step instructions cover today's best approaches, while 245 crisp illustrations demonstrate relevant anatomy, insertion sites, and nuances of technique. Clinical pearls in each chapter equip you to perform every technique like an expert. **CPT-2000 coding information throughout the text helps you to achieve proper reimbursement.**

Atlas of Common Pain Syndromes   ISBN 0-7216-9211-7

As a companion text to Dr. Waldman's *Uncommon Pain Syndromes*, this all-color atlas examines the diagnosis, evaluation, and treatment of common pain problems. Inside you'll find **ICD-9** diagnosis codes, as well as clinical pearls gleaned from years of professional pain management practice. Over 200 specially created **full-color** drawings—many of syndromes not illustrated in other texts—clarify key concepts. **A wealth of radiographs and CT and MRI scans help you to define each disease entity.**

Atlas of
Uncommon
Pain
Syndromes

Steven D. Waldman, M.D., J.D.
Director
    Pain Consortium of Greater Kansas City
    Leawood, Kansas
Clinical Professor of Anesthesiology
    University of Missouri at Kansas City
    School of Medicine
    Kansas City, Missouri

Illustrations by
Caitlin H. Duckwall
Duckwall Productions
Baltimore, Maryland

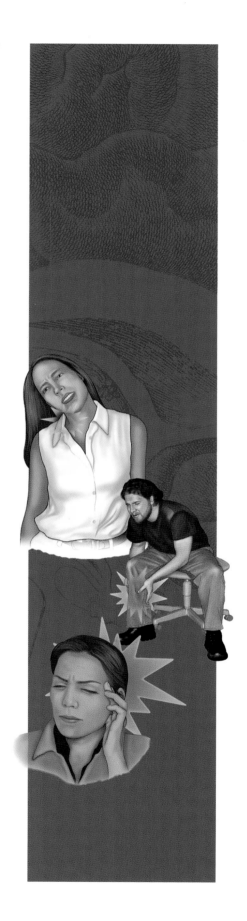

SAUNDERS
An Imprint of Elsevier Science
Philadelphia   London   New York   St. Louis   Sydney   Toronto

SAUNDERS
An Imprint of Elsevier Science

The Curtis Center
Independence Square West
Philadephia, PA 19106

ATLAS OF UNCOMMON PAIN SYNDROMES   ISBN 0-7216-9372-5

Notice

Medicine is an ever-changing field. Standard safety precautions must be followed, but as new research and clinical experience broaden our knowledge, changes in treatment and drug therapy may become necessary or appropriate. Readers are advised to check the most current product information provided by the manufacturer of each drug to be administered to verify the recommended dose, the method and duration of administration, and contraindications. It is the responsibility of the treating physician, relying on experience and knowledge of the patient, to determine dosages and the best treatment for each individual patient. Neither the Publisher nor the editor assumes any liability for any injury and/or damage to persons or property arising from this publication.

The Publisher

Library of Congress Cataloging-in-Publication Data

Atlas of uncommon pain syndromes / editor, Steven D. Waldman; illustrations by Caitlin H. Duckwall.—1st ed.
   p. cm.
     Includes index.
     ISBN 0-7216-9372-5
   1. Pain—Atlases. 2. Syndromes—Atlases. I. Waldman, Steven D.
     RB127 .A88 2003
616'.0472–dc21

                      2002021799

Acquisitions Editor: Allan Ross
Developmental Editor: Arlene Chappelle
Project Manager: Linda Lewis Grigg
Designer: Steven Stave

BS/DNP

Printed in Hong Kong.

Last digit is the print number: 9 8 7 6 5 4 3 2 1

To Judith Tharp, M.D.
Mentor, teacher, and, most important, friend.

Preface

We are all admonished by our medical school professors that *"when you hear hoof beats, think of horses, not zebras."* While in general this is good advice, those of us fortunate enough to have practiced medicine for more than a few years recognize that on occasion, the hoof beats turn out not to be horses . . . and, occasionally, not even zebras. It is this basic truth of medicine that serves as the impetus for writing *Atlas of Uncommon Pain Syndromes.*

In a busy pain management practice, rarely a week goes by that I or one of my colleagues is not challenged by a "zebra." Two things are consistent about most of these unique or unusual cases: (1) by and large, the patients were seen by caring and conscientious physicians who simply failed to think of the "zebras" hidden in the patient's clinical presentation; and (2) in retrospect, the unusual or unique diagnosis was usually obvious once it was elucidated. That is not to say that any of us are always able to identify the "zebras." Many times, it is the next doctor in line to see the patient who is able to put all the pieces together and make the correct diagnosis.

In *Atlas of Uncommon Pain Syndromes,* I have tried to identify the "zebras" that seem to elude us with sufficient frequency to make taking a focused look at them more than an exercise in academic snobbery. I have endeavored to pick real diagnoses, rather than exotic or rare diseases or uncommon manifestations of common diseases. In another words, I have tried to provide clinicians with information that will help them help their patients. Beautiful full-color artwork by Caitlin Duckwall helps highlight the common pathopneumonic features of each disease, making it easier for the clinician to remember them. ICD-9 codes are provided for each diagnosis to help the clinician get paid for the work he or she does. A section on clinical pearls is also presented for each diagnosis to provide practical—and sometimes hard-to-find—information on how to best care for patients suffering from these unique and unusual diseases.

I hope that you enjoy reading *Atlas of Uncommon Pain Syndromes* as much as I enjoyed writing it.

Steven D. Waldman

Contents

I

Headache Pain Syndromes

1 Ice Pick Headache

ICD-9 CODE 784.0

THE CLINICAL SYNDROME

Ice pick headache is a constellation of symptoms consisting of paroxysms of stabbing jabs and jolts that occur primarily in the first division of the trigeminal nerve. These paroxysms of pain may occur as a single jab or a series of jabs that last for a fraction of a second followed by relatively pain-free episodes. The pain of ice pick headache occurs in irregular intervals of hours to days. Like cluster headache, ice pick headache is an episodic disorder that is characterized by "clusters" of painful attacks followed by pain-free periods. Episodes of ice pick headache usually occur on the same side, but in rare patients, the pain may move to the same anatomic region on the contralateral side. Ice pick headache occurs more commonly in women and is generally not seen before the fourth decade of life, but rare reports of children suffering from ice pick headache sporadically appear in the literature. Synonyms for ice pick headache include *jabs and jolts headache* and *idiopathic stabbing headache.*

SIGNS AND SYMPTOMS

The patient suffering from ice pick headache complains of jolts or jabs of pain in the orbit, temple, or parietal region (Fig. 1–1). Some patients describe the pain of ice pick headache as a sudden smack or slap on the side of the head. Like patients suffering from trigeminal neuralgia, the patient suffering from ice pick headache may exhibit involuntary muscle spasms of the affected area in response to the paroxysms of pain. In contradistinction to trigeminal neuralgia, which involves the first division of the trigeminal nerve, there are no trigger areas that induce the pain of ice pick headache. The neurological examination of a patient suffering from ice pick headache is normal. Some patients exhibit anxiety and depression because the intensity of pain associated with ice pick headache leads many patients to believe they are suffering from a brain tumor.

TESTING

Magnetic resonance imaging (MRI) of the brain provides the clinician with the best information regarding the cranial vault and its contents. MRI is highly accurate and helps to identify abnormalities that may put the patient at risk for neurological disasters due to intracranial and brainstem pathology, including tumors and demyelinating disease. Magnetic resonance angiography (MRA) may also be useful in helping identify aneurysms, which may be responsible for the patient's neurological findings. In patients who cannot undergo MRI scanning, such as a patient with a pacemaker, computed tomography is a reasonable second choice. Radionuclide bone scanning and plain radiography are indicated if fracture or bony abnormality such as metastatic disease is considered in the differential diagnosis.

Screening laboratory testing consisting of complete blood cell count, erythrocyte sedimentation rate, and automated blood chemistry testing should be performed if the diagnosis of ice pick headache is in question. Measurement of intraocular pressure should be performed if glaucoma is suspected.

DIFFERENTIAL DIAGNOSIS

Ice pick headache is a clinical diagnosis that is supported by a combination of clinical history, normal physical examination, radiography, and MRI. Pain syndromes that may mimic ice pick headache include trigeminal neuralgia involving the first division of the trigeminal nerve, demyelinating disease, and chronic paroxysmal hemicrania. Trigeminal neuralgia involving the first division of the trigeminal

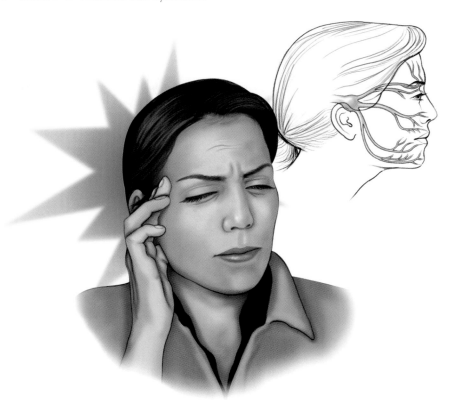

Figure 1-1. Ice pick headache is characterized by jabs or jolts in the orbit, temple, or parietal region.

nerve is uncommon and is characterized by trigger areas and tic-like movements. Demyelinating disease is generally associated with other neurological findings, including optic neuritis and other motor and sensory abnormalities. The pain of chronic paroxysmal hemicrania lasts much longer than the pain of ice pick headache and is associated with redness and watering of the ipsilateral eye.

TREATMENT

Ice pick headache uniformly responds to treatment with indomethacin. In fact, failure to respond to indomethacin puts the diagnosis of ice pick headache in question. A starting dosage of 25 mg daily for 2 days titrating upward to 25 mg three times a day is a reasonable treatment approach. This dose may be carefully increased up to 150 mg per day. Indomethacin must be used carefully, if at all, in patients with peptic ulcer disease or impaired renal function. Anecdotal reports of a positive response to the cyclooxygenase-2 inhibitors in the treatment of ice pick headache have been noted in the headache literature. Underlying sleep disturbance and depression are best treated with a tricylic antidepressant compound such as nortriptyline, which can be started at a single bedtime dose of 25 mg.

COMPLICATIONS AND SIDE EFFECTS

Failure to correctly diagnosis ice pick headache may put the patient at risk if intracranial pathology or demyelinating disease, which may mimic the clinical presentation of chronic paroxysmal hemicrania, is overlooked. MRI is indicated in all patients thought to be suffering from ice pick headache. Failure to diagnose glaucoma, which may also cause intermittent ocular pain, may result in permanent loss of sight.

CLINICAL PEARLS

The diagnosis of ice pick headache is made by taking a careful targeted headache history. Patients suffering from ice pick headache should have a normal neurological examination. If the results of the neurological examination are abnormal, the diagnosis of ice pick headache should be discarded and a careful search for the cause of the patient's neurological findings undertaken.

2 Chronic Paroxysmal Hemicrania

ICD-9 CODE 784.0

THE CLINICAL SYNDROME

Chronic paroxysmal hemicrania shares many characteristics of its more common analogue cluster headache but has several important differences (Table 2–1). Like cluster headache, chronic paroxysmal hemicrania is a severe, episodic, unilateral headache that affects the periorbital and retro-orbital regions. Unlike cluster headaches, which occurs 10 times more commonly in males, chronic paroxysmal hemicrania occurs primarily in females. The duration of pain associated with chronic paroxysmal hemicrania is shorter than that of cluster headache, lasting from 5 to 45 minutes. This pain does not follow the chronobiological pattern seen in cluster headache sufferers. Patients with chronic paroxysmal hemicrania will usually experience more than five attacks per day. Chronic paroxysmal hemicrania uniformly responds to indomethacin, whereas cluster headache does not.

SIGNS AND SYMPTOMS

During attacks of chronic paroxysmal hemicrania, patients exhibit the following physical findings suggestive of a Horner's syndrome on the ipsilateral side of the pain (Fig. 2–1).
- Conjunctival and scleral injection
- Lacrimation
- Nasal congestion
- Rhinorrhea
- Ptosis of the eyelid

As in cluster headache, the patient may become agitated during attacks rather than seeking dark and quiet as does the migraneur. Unlike cluster headache, alcohol does not appear to trigger attacks of chronic paroxysmal hemicrania. Between attacks, the neuro-logical examination of the patient suffering from chronic paroxysmal hemicrania should be normal.

TESTING

Magnetic resonance imaging (MRI) of the brain provides the clinician with the best information regarding the cranial vault and its contents. MRI is highly accurate and helps to identify abnormalities that may put the patient at risk for neurological disasters due to intracranial and brainstem pathology, including tumors and demyelinating disease. Magnetic resonance angiography may also be useful in helping identify aneurysms, which may be responsible for the patient's neurological findings. In patients who cannot undergo MRI scanning, such as a patient with a pacemaker, computed tomography is a reasonable second choice. Radionuclide bone scanning and plain radiography are indicated if fracture or bony abnormality such as metastatic disease is considered in the differential diagnosis.

Screening laboratory testing consisting of complete blood cell count, erythrocyte sedimentation rate, and automated blood chemistry testing should be performed if the diagnosis of chronic paroxysmal

Table 2–1. Comparison of Cluster Headache and Chronic Paroxysmal Hemicrania

	Cluster Headache	Chronic Paroxysmal Hemicrania
Gender	Predominately male	Predominately female
Response to Indomethacin	Negative	Positive
Chronobiological pattern	Positive	Negative
Alcohol trigger	Positive	Negative
Length of attacks	Longer	Shorter
Horner's syndrome	Present	Present

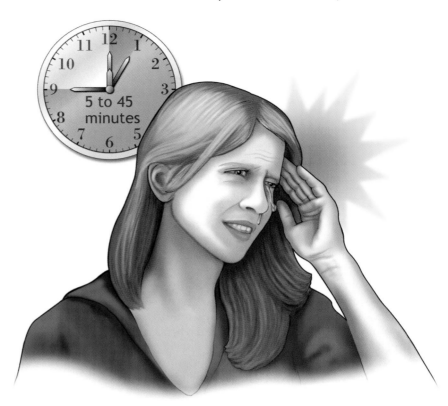

Figure 2–1. Unlike cluster headache, which occurs primarily in males, chronic paroxysmal hemicrania occurs primarily in females.

hemicrania is in question. Measurement of intra-ocular pressure should be performed if glaucoma is suspected.

DIFFERENTIAL DIAGNOSIS

Chronic paroxysmal hemicrania is a clinical diagnosis that is supported by a combination of clinical history, abnormal physical examination during attacks, radiography, and MRI. Pain syndromes that may mimic chronic paroxysmal hemicrania include cluster headache, trigeminal neuralgia involving the first division of the trigeminal nerve, demyelinating disease, and ice pick headache. Trigeminal neuralgia involving the first division of the trigeminal nerve is uncommon and is characterized by trigger areas and tic-like movements. Demyelinating disease is generally associated with other neurological findings, including optic neuritis and other motor and sensory abnormalities. The pain of cluster headache lasts much longer than does the pain of chronic paroxysmal hemicrania and has a male predominance, a chronobiological pattern of attacks, and a lack of response to treatment with indomethacin.

TREATMENT

Chronic paroxysmal hemicrania uniformly responds to treatment with indomethacin. In fact, failure to respond to indomethacin puts the diagnosis of chronic paroxysmal hemicrania in question. A starting dose of 25 mg daily for 2 days titrating upward to 25 mg three times a day is a reasonable treatment approach. This dose may be carefully increased up to 150 mg per day. Indomethacin must be used carefully, if at all, in patients with peptic ulcer disease or impaired renal function. Anecdotal reports of a positive response to the cyclooxygenase-2 (COX-2) inhibitors in the treatment of chronic paroxysmal hemicrania have been noted in the headache literature. Underlying sleep disturbance and depression are best treated with a tricylic antidepressant compound such as nortriptyline, which can be started at a single bedtime dose of 25 mg.

COMPLICATIONS AND SIDE EFFECTS

A failure to correctly diagnose chronic paroxysmal hemicrania may put the patient at risk if intracranial pathology or demyelinating disease that may mimic the clinical presentation of chronic paroxysmal hemicrania is overlooked. MRI scanning is indicated in all patients thought to be suffering from chronic paroxysmal hemicrania. Failure to diagnose glaucoma, which may also cause intermittent ocular pain, may result in permanent loss of sight.

CLINICAL PEARLS

The diagnosis of chronic paroxysmal hemicrania is made by taking a careful targeted headache history. Between attacks, patients suffering from chronic paroxysmal hemicrania should have a normal neurological examination. If the neurological examination is abnormal between attacks, the diagnosis of chronic paroxysmal hemicrania should be discarded and a careful search for the cause of the patient's neurological findings undertaken.

3 Sexual Headache

ICD-9 CODE 784.0

THE CLINICAL SYNDROME

Sexual headache is a term used to describe a group of headaches associated with sexual history. Clinicians have identified three general types of headache associated with sexual activity

- Explosive type
- Dull type
- Postural type

Each of these sexual headache types was previously called *benign coital headache,* but this term has been replaced by sexual headache because each may occur with sexual activity other than coitus (Fig. 3–1). In general, sexual headache includes a benign group of disorders, but a rare patient may suffer acute subarachnoid hemorrhage during sexual activity, which may be erroneously diagnosed as benign explosive-type sexual headache. There is no gender predilection for sexual headache, and the occurrence of all types of sexual headache may be episodic rather than chronic in nature. Rarely, more than one type of sexual headache occurs in the same patient.

SIGNS AND SYMPTOMS

The patient suffering from sexual headache presents differently depending on the type of sexual headache he or she suffers from. Each clinical presentation is discussed below.

Explosive-Type Sexual Headache

Explosive-type sexual headache is the most common type of sexual headache encountered in clinical practice. The patient usually presents to the clinician fearing he or she has had a stroke. The patient may be less forthcoming about the circum-

stances surrounding the onset of headache, and tactful questioning may be required to ascertain the actual clinical history. Explosive-type sexual headache occurs suddenly with an almost instantaneous onset to peak just before or during orgasm. The intensity of explosive-type sexual headache is severe and has been likened to the pain of acute subarachnoid hemorrhage. The location of pain is usually occipital, but some patients volunteer that the pain felt "like the top of my head was going to blow off." The pain is usually bilateral, but there are isolated reports of unilateral explosive-type sexual headache. The pain usually remains intense for 10 to 15 minutes and then gradually abates. Some patients note some residual headache pain for up to 2 days.

Dull-Type Sexual Headache

Dull-type sexual headache begins during the early portion of sexual activity. This headache type is aching in character and begins in the occipital region. The headache becomes holocranial as sexual activity progresses toward orgasm. It may peak at orgasm, but unlike explosive-type headache, dull-type sexual headache disappears rapidly after orgasm. Ceasing sexual activity usually aborts dull-type sexual headache. Some headache specialists believe that dull-type sexual headache is simply a milder version of explosive-type sexual headache.

Postural-Type Sexual Headache

Postural-type sexual headache is similar to explosive-type sexual headache in that it occurs just before or during orgasm. Its rapid onset to peak and severe intensity are also similar to explosive-type headache. It differs from explosive-type headache in that the headache symptoms recur when the patient stands up, in a manner analogous to postdural puncture headache. The postural component of this type

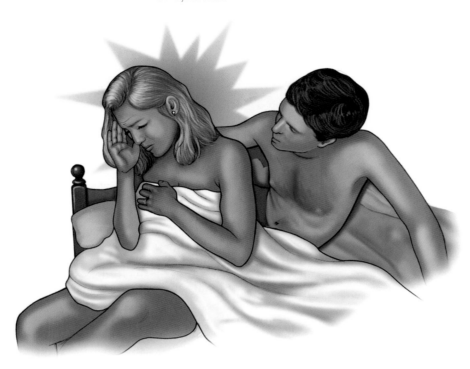

Figure 3-1. Sexual headaches show no gender predilection and are generally benign in nature.

of sexual headache is thought to be due to minute tears in the dura that occur during intense sexual activity.

TESTING

Magnetic resonance imaging (MRI) of the brain provides the clinician with the best information regarding the cranial vault and its contents. MRI is highly accurate and helps to identify abnormalities that may put the patient at risk for neurological disasters due to intracranial and brainstem pathology, including tumors and demyelinating disease. More important, MRI helps to identify bleeding associated with leaking intracranial aneurysms. Magnetic resonance angiography (MRA) may be useful to help identify aneurysms responsible for the patient's neurological symptomatology. In patients who cannot undergo MRI, such as a patient with a pacemaker, computed tomography (CT) scanning is a reasonable second choice. Even if blood is not present on MRI or CT, if intracranial hemorrhage is suspected, lumbar puncture should be performed.

Screening laboratory testing consisting of complete blood cell count, erythrocyte sedimentation rate, and automated blood chemistry testing should be performed if the diagnosis of sexual headache is in question. Measurement of intraocular pressure should be performed if glaucoma is suspected.

DIFFERENTIAL DIAGNOSIS

Sexual headache is a clinical diagnosis that is supported by a combination of clinical history, normal physical examination, radiography, MRI, and MRA. Pain syndromes that may mimic sexual headache include trigeminal neuralgia involving the first division of the trigeminal nerve, demyelinating disease, cluster headache, migraine, and chronic paroxysmal hemicrania. Trigeminal neuralgia involving the first division of the trigeminal nerve is uncommon and is characterized by trigger areas and tic-like movements. Demyelinating disease is generally associated with other neurological findings, including optic neuritis and other motor and sensory abnormalities. The pain of chronic paroxysmal hemicrania and cluster is associated with redness and watering of the ipsilateral eye, nasal congestion, and rhinorrhea during the headache. These findings are absent in all types of sexual headache. Migraine headache may or may not be associated with nonpainful neurological findings known as *aura,* but the patient will almost always report some systemic symptoms, such as nausea or photophobia, not typically associated with sexual headache.

TREATMENT

It is generally believed that avoiding the inciting activity for a few weeks decreases the propensity to trigger sexual headaches. If this avoidance technique fails or is impractical due to patient preference, a trial of propranolol is a reasonable next step. A low dose of 20 to 40 mg as a daily dose titrating upward in 20-mg steps to 200 mg as a divided daily dose until prophylaxis occurs will treat the vast majority of patients suffering from sexual headache. Propranolol should be used with caution in patients with asthma or cardiac failure as well as those with brittle diabetes.

If propranolol is ineffective, indomethacin may be tried. A starting dose of 25 mg daily for 2 days titrating upward to 25 mg three times a day is a reasonable treatment approach. This dose may be carefully increased up to 150 mg per day. Indomethacin must be used carefully, if at all, in patients with peptic ulcer disease or impaired renal function. Anecdotal reports of a positive response to the cyclooxygenase-2 (COX-2) inhibitors in the treatment of sexual headache have been noted in the headache literature. Underlying sleep disturbance and depression are best treated with a tricylic antidepressant compound such as nortriptyline, which can be started at a single bedtime dose of 25 mg.

COMPLICATIONS AND SIDE EFFECTS

Failure to correctly diagnosis sexual headache may put the patient at risk if intracranial pathology or demyelinating disease (which may mimic the clinical presentation of sexual headache) is overlooked. MRI and MRA are indicated in all patients thought to be suffering from sexual headache. Failure to diagnose glaucoma, which may also cause intermittent ocular pain, may result in permanent loss of sight.

CLINICAL PEARLS

The diagnosis of sexual headache is made by taking a careful targeted headache history. As mentioned earlier, patients may be less than forthcoming about the events surrounding the onset of their headache, and the clinician should be sensitive to this fact. Patients suffering from sexual headache should have a normal neurological examination. If the neurological examination is abnormal, the diagnosis of sexual headache should be discarded and a careful search for the cause of the patient's neurological findings undertaken.

4

Cough Headache

ICD-9 CODE 784.0

THE CLINICAL SYNDROME

Cough headache is a term used to describe headaches that are triggered by coughing and other activities that are associated with a Valsalva maneuver, such as laughing, straining at stool, lifting, and bending the head toward the ground (Fig. 4–1). Clinicians have identified two types of cough headache.

■ Benign
■ Symptomatic

Initially, both types of cough headache were thought to be related to sexual and exertional headaches, but they are now considered to be distinct clinical entities. There is a strong male predilection for benign cough headache and no gender predilection for symptomatic cough headache.

SIGNS AND SYMPTOMS

The patient suffering from cough headache presents differently depending on the type of cough headache he or she suffers from. Each clinical presentation will be discussed.

Benign Cough Headache

Benign cough headache is associated with no obvious neurological or musculoskeletal disease. More than 80% of patients suffering from benign cough headache are male, in contradistinction to symptomatic cough headache, in which there is no gender predilection. The onset of benign cough headache is abrupt, occurring immediately after coughing or other activities that cause a Valsalva maneuver. Although the intensity of pain is severe and peaks rapidly, it lasts only seconds to minutes.

The character of the pain associated with benign cough headache is splitting or sharp and is located in the occipital region bilaterally and, occasionally, the vertex of the skull. There are no accompanying neurological or systemic symptoms as with cluster and migraine headache. The age of onset of benign cough headache is generally in the late fifth or sixth decade of life. If such headaches occur before the age of 50, there should be strong clinical suspicion that the patient is either suffering from symptomatic cough headache or has pathology in the posterior fossa, such as Arnold-Chiari malformation or tumor, that is responsible for the headache. Tumors of the foramen magnum may also mimic the presentation of benign cough headache if no neurological symptoms are present.

Symptomatic Cough Headache

Symptomatic cough headache is almost always associated with structural abnormalities of the cranium such as Arnold-Chiari malformation or intracranial tumors (Fig. 4–2). The symptomatology associated with symptomatic cough headache is thought to be due to herniation of the cerebellar tonsil through the foramen magnum into the space normally occupied by the upper portion of the cervical spinal cord. Like benign cough headache, the onset of pain associated with symptomatic cough headache is abrupt, occurring immediately after coughing or other activities that cause a Valsalva maneuver. Although the intensity of pain is severe and peaks rapidly, it lasts only seconds to minutes. However, unlike benign cough headache, there may be associated neurological symptoms including difficulty swallowing, faintness, and numbness in the face and upper extremities. These associated symptoms should be taken very seriously because they are indicative of increased intracranial pressure and herniation of the intracranial contents.

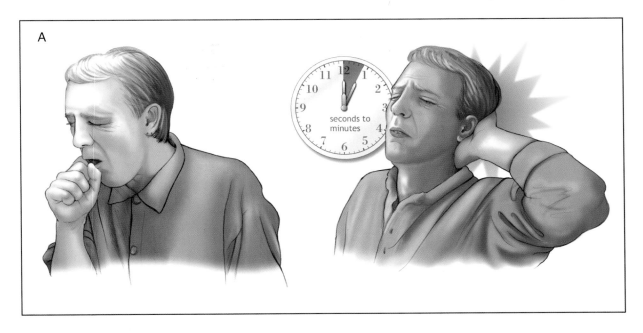

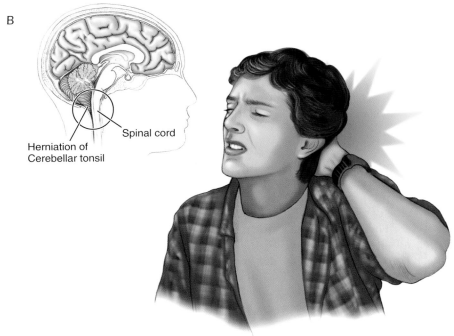

Figure 4–1. *A*, Benign cough headache rarely occurs before the age of 50. *B*, Symptomatic cough headache is often associated with structural abnormalities such as Arnold-Chiari malformation.

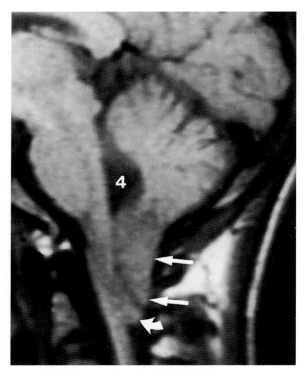

Figure 4–2. Low-lying cerebellar tonsils (*straight arrows*) of a Chiari malformation are shown deforming the medulla (*curved arrow*) in a sagittal T1-weighted SE image. 4, Fourth ventricle. (From Stark DD, Bradley WG Jr [eds]: Magnetic Resonance Imaging, Vol III, 3rd ed. St Louis, Mosby, 1999.)

The character of the pain associated with symptomatic cough headache is splitting or sharp and is located in the occipital region bilaterally and, occasionally, the vertex of the skull. The age of onset of symptomatic cough headache is generally in the third decade of life, although, depending on the amount of neurological compromise, it may occur at any age. Unlike benign cough headache, which occurs predominantly in males, symptomatic cough headache occurs with equal prevalence in both genders.

TESTING

Magnetic resonance imaging (MRI) of the brain provides the clinician with the best information regarding the cranial vault and its contents. MRI is highly accurate and helps to identify abnormalities that may put the patient at risk for neurological disasters due to intracranial and brainstem pathology, including tumors and demyelinating disease. Special attention to the foramen magnum may help identify more subtle abnormalities responsible for posterior fossa neurological signs and symptoms. MRI helps to identify bleeding associated with leaking intracranial

aneurysms, which may mimic the symptoms of both types of cough headache. Magnetic resonance angiography (MRA) may be useful to help identify aneurysms responsible for the patient's neurological symptomatology. In patients who cannot undergo MRI, such as a patient with a pacemaker, computed tomography (CT) is a reasonable second choice. Even if blood is not present on MRI or CT, if intracranial hemorrhage is suspected, lumbar puncture should be performed. Plain radiographs of the cervical spine may also be useful in the evaluation of Arnold-Chiari malformations and should be included in the evaluation of all patients suffering from cough headache.

Screening laboratory testing consisting of complete blood cell count, erythrocyte sedimentation rate, and automated blood chemistry testing should be performed if the diagnosis of cough headache is in question. Measurement of intraocular pressure should be performed if glaucoma is suspected.

DIFFERENTIAL DIAGNOSIS

Cough headache is a clinical diagnosis that is supported by a combination of clinical history, physical examination, radiography, MRI, and MRA. Pain syndromes that may mimic cough headache include benign exertional headache, ice pick headache, sexual headache, trigeminal neuralgia involving the first division of the trigeminal nerve, demyelinating disease, cluster headache, and chronic paroxysmal hemicrania. Trigeminal neuralgia involving the first division of the trigeminal nerve is uncommon and is characterized by trigger areas and tic-like movements. Demyelinating disease is generally associated with other neurological findings, including optic neuritis and other motor and sensory abnormalities. The pain of chronic paroxysmal hemicrania and cluster is associated with redness and watering of the ipsilateral eye, nasal congestion, and rhinorrhea during the headache. These findings are absent in all types of cough headache. Migraine headache may or may not be associated with nonpainful neurological findings known as *aura*, but the patient will almost always report some systemic symptoms, such as nausea or photophobia, not typically associated with cough headache.

TREATMENT

Indomethacin is the treatment of choice for benign cough headache. A starting dose of 25 mg daily for 2 days titrating upward to 25 mg three times a day is a reasonable treatment approach. This dose may be carefully increased up to 150 mg per day. Indomethacin must be used carefully, if at all, in patients with peptic ulcer disease or impaired renal function. Anecdotal reports of a positive response to the cyclooxygenase (COX-2) inhibitors in the treatment of benign cough headache have been noted by headache specialists. Underlying sleep disturbance and depression are best treated with a tricylic antidepressant compound such as nortriptyline, which can be started at a single bedtime dose of 25 mg.

The only uniformly effective treatment for symptomatic cough headache is surgical decompression of the foramen magnum. This is usually accomplished via suboccipital craniectomy. Surgical decompression prevents the low-lying cerebellar tonsils from obstructing the flow of spinal fluid from the cranium to the spinal subarachnoid space during a Valsalva maneuver.

COMPLICATIONS AND SIDE EFFECTS

Failure to correctly diagnosis cough headache may put the patient at risk if intracranial pathology or demyelinating disease (which may mimic the clinical presentation of cough headache) is overlooked. MRI and MRA are indicated in all patients thought to be suffering from cough headache. Failure to diagnose glaucoma, which may also cause intermittent ocular pain, may result in permanent loss of sight.

CLINICAL PEARLS

Any patient presenting with headaches associated with exertion or Valsalva should be taken very seriously. Although statistically most of these headaches will ultimately be proved to be of benign etiology, a small subset of these patients will have potentially life-threatening disease. The diagnosis of cough headache is made by taking a careful targeted headache history and performing a careful physical examination. The clinician must separate those patients suffering from benign cough headache from those suffering from symptomatic cough headache. Patients suffering from benign cough headache should have a normal neurological examination. If the neurological examination is abnormal, the diagnosis of benign cough headache should be discarded and a careful search for the cause of the patient's neurological findings undertaken.

5
Headache Associated with Temporal Arteritis

ICD-9 CODE 446.5

THE CLINICAL SYNDROME

As the name suggests, the headache associated with temporal arteritis is located primarily in the temples, with secondary pain often located in the frontal and occipital regions. A disease of the sixth decade and beyond, temporal arteritis affects whites almost exclusively, and there is a female gender predominance of 3:1. Temporal arteritis is also known as *giant cell arteritis* because of the finding of giant multinucleated cells that infiltrate arteries containing elastin, including the temporal, ophthalmic, and external carotid arteries (Fig. 5–1A). Approximately half of patients with temporal arteritis also suffer from polymyalgia rheumatica.

SIGNS AND SYMPTOMS

Headache is seen in the vast majority of patients suffering from temporal arteritis. The headache is located in the temples and is usually continuous. The character of the headache pain associated with temporal arteritis is aching in nature with a mild to moderate level of intensity. The patient suffering from temporal arteritis may also complain of soreness of the scalp, making the combing of hair or laying on a firm pillow extremely uncomfortable.

Although temporal headache is present in almost all patients suffering from temporal arteritis, it is the finding of intermittent jaw claudication that is pathognomonic for the disease (see Fig. 5–1B). In the elderly patient, jaw pain while chewing should be considered to be secondary to temporal arteritis until proved otherwise. If there is a strong clinical suspicion that the patient has temporal arteritis, immediate treatment with corticosteroids is indicated (see

Treatment). The reason for the need for immediate treatment is the potential for sudden painless deterioration of vision in one eye secondary to ischemia of the optic nerve.

In addition to the signs and symptoms mentioned, patients suffering from temporal arteritis experience myalgia and morning stiffness. Muscle weakness associated with inflammatory muscle disease and many of the other collagen vascular diseases is absent in temporal arteritis unless the patient has been treated with prolonged doses of corticosteroids for other systemic disease, such as polymyalgia rheumatica. The patient may also experience nonspecific systemic symptoms including malaise, weight loss, night sweats, and depression.

On physical examination, a swollen, indurated, nodular temporal artery is present. Diminished pulses are often noted, as is tenderness to palpation. Scalp tenderness to palpation is often seen. Funduscopic examination may reveal a pale, edematous optic disc. The patient suffering from temporal arteritis often appears chronically ill, depressed, or both.

TESTING

Erythrocyte sedimentation rate testing should be obtained on all patients suspected of having temporal arteritis. In temporal arteritis, the erythrocyte sedimentation rate is greater than 50 mm/hr in more than 90% of patients. Less than 2% of patients with biopsy-proven temporal arteritis have normal erythrocyte sedimentation rates. Ideally, the blood for the erythrocyte sedimentation rate should be obtained before beginning corticosteroid therapy because the initial level of elevation of this test is useful not only to help diagnose the disease but also as a mechanism to establish the efficacy of therapy. It is important for the clinician to remember that the erythrocyte sedimentation rate is a nonspecific test and that other diseases that may present clinically in a manner similar to temporal arteritis, such as malig-

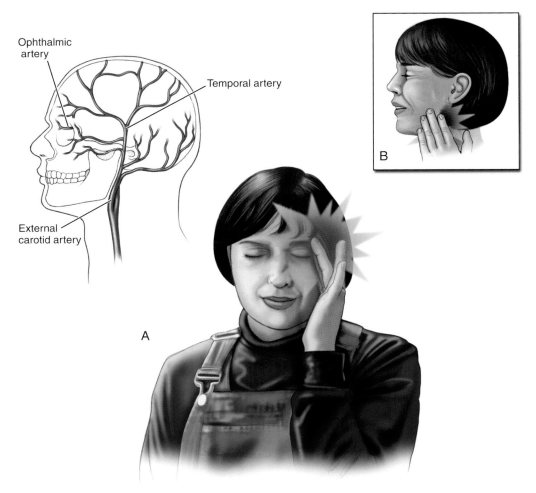

Figure 5–1. *A,* Temporal arteritis is a disease of the sixth decade that occurs almost exclusively in whites, with a predilection of 3:1 for women. *B,* The sine qua non of temporal arteritis is jaw claudication.

nancy or infection, may also markedly elevate the erythrocyte sedimentation rate. Therefore, confirmation of the clinical diagnosis of temporal arteritis requires a temporal artery biopsy.

Given the simplicity and safety of temporal artery biopsy, this test should probably be performed on all patients suspected of suffering from temporal arteritis. The presence of an inflammatory infiltrate with giant cells in the biopsied artery is characteristic of the disease. Edema of the intima and disruption of the internal elastic lamina strengthen the diagnosis. A small percentage of patients with clinical signs and symptoms strongly suggestive of temporal arteritis who also exhibit a significantly elevated erythrocyte sedimentation rate will have a negative temporal artery biopsy. As mentioned, if there is a strong clinical impression that the patient in fact has temporal arteritis, an immediate blood sample for erythrocyte sedimentation rate testing should be obtained and the patient started on corticosteroids. Complete blood cell count and automated chemistries including thyroid testing are indicated in all patients with suspected temporal arteritis to help rule out other systemic disease that may mimic the clinical presentation of temporal arteritis.

If the diagnosis of temporal arteritis is in doubt, magnetic resonance imaging (MRI) of the brain provides the clinician with the best information regarding the cranial vault and its contents. MRI is highly accurate and helps to identify abnormalities that may put the patient at risk for neurological disasters due to intracranial and brainstem pathology, including tumors and demyelinating disease. More important, MRI helps to identify bleeding associated with leaking intracranial aneurysms. Magnetic resonance angiography may be useful to help identify aneurysms responsible for the patient's neurological symptomatology. In patients who cannot undergo MRI, such as a patient with a pacemaker, computed tomography (CT) scanning is a reasonable second choice. Even if blood is not present on MRI or CT, if intracranial hemorrhage is suspected, lumbar puncture should be performed. Measurement of intraocular pressure should be performed if glaucoma is suspected.

DIFFERENTIAL DIAGNOSIS

Headache associated with temporal arteritis is a clinical diagnosis that is supported by a combination of clinical history, abnormal physical examination of the temporal artery, normal radiography, MRI, an elevated erythrocyte sedimentation rate, and a positive temporal artery biopsy. Pain syndromes that may mimic temporal arteritis include tension-type headache, brain tumor, other forms of arteritis,

trigeminal neuralgia involving the first division of the trigeminal nerve, demyelinating disease, migraine headache, cluster headache, migraine, and chronic paroxysmal hemicrania. Trigeminal neuralgia involving the first division of the trigeminal nerve is uncommon and is characterized by trigger areas and tic-like movements. Demyelinating disease is generally associated with other neurological findings, including optic neuritis and other motor and sensory abnormalities. The pain of chronic paroxysmal hemicrania and cluster is associated with redness and watering of the ipsilateral eye, nasal congestion, and rhinorrhea during the headache. These findings are absent in all types of sexual headache. Migraine headache may or may not be associated with nonpainful neurological findings known as *aura,* but the patient almost always reports some systemic symptoms, such as nausea or photophobia, not typically associated with the headache of temporal arteritis.

TREATMENT

The mainstay of the treatment of temporal arteritis and its associated headaches and other systemic symptoms is the immediate use of corticosteroids. If visual symptoms are present, an initial dose of 80 mg of prednisone is indicated. This dose should be continued until the symptoms of temporal arteritis have completely abated. At this point, the dose may be decreased by 5 mg/wk as long as the symptoms remain quiescent and the erythrocyte sedimentation rate does not rise. Consideration of cytoprotection of the stomach mucosa should be given because the possibility of ulceration and gastrointestinal bleeding remains a real problem. If the patient cannot tolerate the corticosteroids or the maintenance dose of steroids remains so high as to produce adverse effects, azathioprine is a reasonable next choice.

COMPLICATIONS AND SIDE EFFECTS

Failure to promptly recognize, diagnose, and treat temporal arteritis may result in the permanent loss of vision. Failure to correctly diagnose the headache associated with temporal arteritis may put the patient at risk if intracranial pathology or demyelinating disease (which may mimic the clinical presentation of sexual headache) is overlooked. MRI of the brain is indicated in all patients thought to be suffering from headaches associated with temporal arteritis. Failure to diagnose glaucoma, which may also cause intermittent ocular pain, may result in permanent loss of sight.

CLINICAL PEARLS

The diagnosis of headache associated with temporal arteritis is made by taking a careful targeted headache history. As mentioned, jaw claudication is pathognomonic for temporal arteritis, and its presence should be sought in all elderly patients presenting with headache. Failure to promptly recognize, diagnose, and treat temporal arteritis may result in the permanent loss of vision.

6

Post–Dural Puncture Headache

ICD-9 CODE 349.0

THE CLINICAL SYNDROME

Whenever the dura is intentionally or accidentally punctured, the potential for headache exists. The clinical presentation of post–dural puncture headache is classic and makes the diagnosis straightforward if one simply thinks about this diagnostic category of headache. The diagnosis may be obscured if the clinician is unaware that the possibility of dural puncture has occurred or in the rare instance when this type of headache occurs spontaneously after a bout of sneezing or coughing. The etiology of the symptoms and rare physical findings associated with post–dural puncture headache are due to low cerebrospinal fluid pressure resulting from continued leakage of spinal fluid out of the subarachnoid space.

The symptoms of post–dural puncture headache begin almost immediately after the patient moves from a horizontal to an upright position. The intensity peaks within 1 or 2 minutes and abates within several minutes of the patient again assuming the horizontal position. The headache is pounding in character and its intensity is severe, with the intensity increasing the longer the patient remains upright. The headache is almost always bilateral and located in the frontal, temporal, and occipital region. Nausea and vomiting as well as dizziness frequently accompany the headache pain, especially if the patient remains upright for long periods. If cranial nerve palsy occurs, visual disturbance may occur.

SIGNS AND SYMPTOMS

The diagnosis of post–dural puncture headache is most often made on the basis of clinical history rather than physical findings on examination. The neuro-logical examination in the vast majority of patients suffering from post–dural puncture headache will be normal. If the spinal fluid leak is allowed to persist or if the patient remains in the upright position for long periods of time despite the headache, cranial nerve palsies may occur, with the sixth cranial nerve affected most commonly. This complication may be transient but may become permanent, especially in patients with vulnerable nerves such as diabetics. If the neurological examination is abnormal, other causes of headache should be considered, including subarachnoid hemorrhage.

The onset of headache pain and other associated symptoms such as nausea and vomiting that appear when the patient moves from the horizontal to the upright position and then abates when the patient resumes a horizontal position is the sine qua non of post–dural puncture headache (Fig. 6–1). A history of intentional dural puncture, such as lumbar puncture, spinal anesthesia, or myelography, or accidental dural puncture, such as failed epidural block or dural injury during spinal surgery, points strongly to the diagnosis of post–dural puncture headache. As mentioned, a spontaneous postural headache that presents identically to headache after dural puncture can occur after bouts of heavy sneezing or coughing and is thought to be due to traumatic rents in the dura. In this setting, a diagnosis of post–dural puncture headache is one of exclusion.

TESTING

Magnetic resonance imaging (MRI) with and without gadolinium are highly accurate in helping confirm the diagnosis of post–dural puncture headache. Enhancement of the dura with low lying cerebellar tonsils will invariably be present. Poor visualization of the cisterns and subdural and epidural fluid collections may also be identified. No additional testing is indicated for the patient who has undergone dural puncture and then develops a

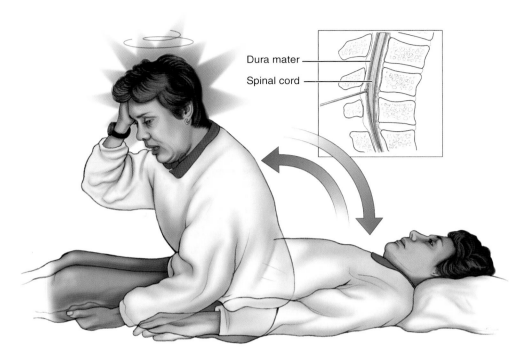

Dura mater
Spinal cord

Figure 6–1. The onset of headache that appears when the patient moves from the horizontal to the upright position is the sine qua non of post–dural puncture headache.

classic postural headache unless infection or sub-arachnoid hemorrhage is suspected. In this setting, lumbar puncture, complete blood cell count, and erythrocyte sedimentation rate are indicated on an emergent basis.

DIFFERENTIAL DIAGNOSIS

If the clinician is aware that the patient has under-gone dural puncture, then the diagnosis of post–dural puncture headache is usually made. It is in those settings in which dural puncture is not sus-pected that delayed diagnosis most often occurs. Occasionally, post–dural puncture is misdiagnosed as migraine headache due to the associated nausea and vomiting coupled with visual disturbance. In any patient with dural puncture, infection remains an ever-present possibility. If fever is present, immedi-ate lumbar puncture and blood cultures should be obtained and the patient started on antibiotics that cover resistant strains of *Staphylococcus.* MRI to rule out epidural abscess should also be considered if fever is present. Subarachnoid hemorrhage may also mimic post–dural puncture headache but should be identified on MRI of the brain.

TREATMENT

The mainstay of the treatment of post–dural punc-ture headache is the administration of autologous blood into the epidural space. This technique is known as *epidural blood patch* and is highly successful in the treatment of post–dural puncture headache. A volume of 12 to 18 mL of autologous blood is injected slowly into the epidural space at the level of dural puncture under strict aseptic precautions. The patient should remain in the horizontal position for the next 12 to 24 hours. Relief will occur within 2 to 3 hours in more than 90% of patients. Approximately 10% of patients will experience temporary relief but will experience a recurrence of symptoms when assuming the upright position. These patients should undergo a second epidural blood patch within 24 hours.

If the patient has experienced significant nausea and vomiting, antiemetics combined with intra-venous fluids will help speed recovery. Some clini-cians have advocated the use of alcoholic beverages to suppress the secretion of antidiuretic hormone and to increase cerebrospinal fluid production. Caffeine has also been reported to be of value in helping to treat the headache pain.

COMPLICATIONS AND SIDE EFFECTS

Failure to promptly recognize, diagnose, and treat post–dural puncture headache may result in consid-erable pain and suffering for the patient. If the low spinal fluid pressure is allowed to persist, cranial nerve deficits may occur. In most instances, the cranial nerve deficits are temporary, but in rare instances, these deficits may become permanent, especially in those patients with vulnerable nerves, such as diabetics. MRI of the brain is indicated in all patients thought to be suffering from headaches asso-ciated with post–dural puncture headache. Failure to correctly diagnose central nervous system infection can result in significant mortality and morbidity.

CLINICAL PEARLS

The diagnosis of headache associated with post–dural puncture is made by taking a careful targeted headache history. The postural nature is pathogno-monic for post–dural puncture headache, and its presence should lead the clinician to strongly con-sider the diagnosis of post–dural puncture headache. The incidence of post–dural puncture after lumbar puncture, myelography, or spinal anesthesia can be decreased by using needles with a smaller dia-meter and placing the needle bevel parallel to the dural fibers. Special noncutting needles may fur-ther decrease the incidence of post–dural puncture headache.

II

Facial Pain Syndromes

7 *Ramsay Hunt Syndrome*

ICD-9 CODE 053.11

THE CLINICAL SYNDROME

Ramsay Hunt syndrome is the eponym given to an acute herpes zoster involving the geniculate ganglion. The syndrome is due to reactivation of the varicella-zoster virus (VZV) within the geniculate ganglion. The VZV is also the causative agent of chickenpox (varicella). Primary infection in the nonimmune host manifests itself clinically as the childhood disease chickenpox. It is postulated that during the course of primary infection with VZV, the virus invades the geniculate ganglia. The virus then remains dormant in the ganglia, producing no clinically evident disease. In some individuals, the virus invades the reactivates and travels along the pathways of the geniculate ganglion, producing the pain and skin lesions characteristic of shingles. The reason that reactivation occurs in only some individuals is not fully understood, but it is theorized that a decrease in cell-mediated immunity may play an important role in the evolution of this disease entity by allowing the virus to multiply in the ganglia and spread to the corresponding sensory nerves, producing clinical disease. Patients who are suffering from malignancies (particularly lymphoma), receiving immunosuppressive therapy (chemotherapy, steroids, radiation), or suffering from chronic diseases are generally debilitated and much more likely than the healthy population to develop acute herpes zoster. These patients all have in common a decreased cell-mediated immune response, which may be the reason for their propensity to develop shingles. This may also explain why the incidence of shingles increases dramatically in patients older than 60 years and is relatively uncommon in persons younger than age 20.

The first division of the trigeminal nerve is the second most common site for the development of acute herpes zoster following the thoracic dermatomes. Rarely, the virus may attack the geniculate ganglion, resulting in facial pain, hearing loss, vertigo, vesicles in the ear, and pain. This constellation of symptoms is called the Ramsay Hunt syndrome and must be distinguished from acute herpes zoster involving the first division of the trigeminal nerve.

SIGNS AND SYMPTOMS

As viral reactivation occurs, ganglionitis and peripheral neuritis cause pain, which is generally localized to the segmental distribution of the geniculate ganglion. This pain may be accompanied by flu-like symptoms and generally progresses from a dull, aching sensation to dysesthetic neuritic pain in the distribution of the geniculate ganglion. In most patients, the pain of acute herpes zoster precedes the eruption of rash by 3 to 7 days, often leading to erroneous diagnosis (see Differential Diagnosis). However, in most patients, the clinical diagnosis of shingles is readily made when the characteristic rash appears. Like chickenpox, the rash of herpes zoster appears in crops of macular lesions, which rapidly progress to papules and then to vesicles (Fig. 7–1). As the disease progresses, the vesicles coalesce and crusting occurs. The area affected by the disease can be extremely painful, and the pain tends to be exacerbated by any movement or contact (e.g., with clothing or sheets). As healing takes place, the crusts fall away, leaving pink scars in the distribution of the rash that gradually become hypopigmented and atrophic.

In most patients, the hyperesthesia and pain generally resolve as the skin lesions heal. In some, however, pain may persist beyond lesion healing. This most common and feared complication of acute herpes zoster is called *postherpetic neuralgia,* and the elderly are affected at a higher rate than the general

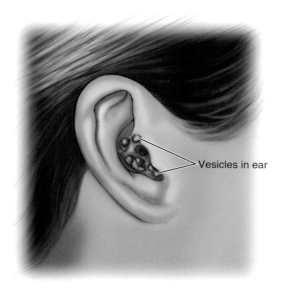

Vesicles in ear

Figure 7–1. Ramsay Hunt syndrome is due to infection of the geniculate ganglion by the varicella-zoster virus.

population suffering from acute herpes zoster. The symptoms of postherpetic neuralgia can vary from a mild self-limited problem to a debilitating, constantly burning pain that is exacerbated by light touch, movement, anxiety, and/or temperature change. This unremitting pain may be so severe that it completely devastates the patient's life and ultimately can lead to suicide. It is the desire to avoid this disastrous sequel to a usually benign self-limited disease that dictates that the clinician use all possible therapeutic efforts for the patient suffering from acute herpes zoster in the geniculate ganglion.

TESTING

Although in most instances the diagnosis of acute herpes zoster involving the geniculate ganglion is easily made of clinical grounds, occasionally, confirmatory testing is required. Such testing may be desirable in patients with other skin lesions that confuse the clinical picture, such as patients with acquired immunodeficiency syndrome who are suffering from Kaposi's sarcoma. In such patients, the diagnosis of acute herpes zoster may be confirmed by obtaining a Tzanck smear from the base of a fresh vesicle, which will reveal multinucleated giant cells and eosinophilic inclusions. To differentiate acute herpes zoster from localized herpes simplex infection, the clinician can obtain fluid from a fresh vesicle and submit it for immunofluorescent testing.

DIFFERENTIAL DIAGNOSIS

Careful initial evaluation, including a thorough history and physical examination, is indicated in all patients suffering from acute herpes zoster involving the geniculate ganglion to rule out occult malignancy or systemic disease that may be responsible for the patient's immunocompromised state and to allow early recognition of changes in clinical status that may presage the development of complications, including myelitis or dissemination of the disease. Other causes of pain in the distribution of the geniculate ganglion include trigeminal neuralgia, sinus disease, glaucoma, retro-orbital tumors and inflammatory diseases such as Tolusa-Hunt syndrome, and intracranial pathology, including tumors.

TREATMENT

The therapeutic challenge of the patient presenting with acute herpes zoster involving the geniculate ganglion is twofold: (1) the immediate relief of acute pain and symptoms and (2) the prevention of complications, including postherpetic neuralgia. It is the consensus of most pain specialists that the earlier in the natural course of the disease that treatment is initiated, the less likely it is that the patient will develop postherpetic neuralgia. Furthermore, because the older patient is at highest risk for developing postherpetic neuralgia early, aggressive treatment of this group of patients is mandatory.

Nerve Blocks

Sympathetic neural blockade with local anesthetics and steroids via stellate ganglion block appears to be the treatment of choice to relieve the symptoms of acute herpes zoster involving the geniculate ganglion as well as to prevent the occurrence of postherpetic neuralgia. Sympathetic nerve block is thought to achieve these goals by blocking the profound sympathetic stimulation that is a result of the viral inflammation of the nerve and geniculate ganglion. If untreated, this sympathetic hyperactivity can cause ischemia secondary to decreased blood flow of the intraneural capillary bed. If this ischemia is allowed to persist, endoneural edema forms, increasing endoneural pressure and causing a further reduction of endoneural blood flow with irreversible nerve damage.

As vesicular crusting occurs, the addition of steroids to the local anesthetic may decrease neural scarring and further decrease the incidence of postherpetic neuralgia. These sympathetic blocks should be continued aggressively until the patient is pain free and should be reimplemented at the return of pain. Failure to use sympathetic neural blockade immediately and aggressively, especially in the elderly, may sentence the patient to a lifetime of suffering from postherpetic neuralgia. Occasionally, some patients suffering from acute herpes zoster involving the geniculate ganglion may not experience pain relief from stellate ganglion block but will respond to blockade of the trigeminal nerve.

Opioid Analgesics

Opioid analgesics may be useful in relieving the aching pain that is often present during the acute stages of herpes zoster as sympathetic nerve blocks are being implemented. They are less effective in the relief of the neuritic pain that is often present. Careful administration of potent, long-acting narcotic analgesics (e.g., oral morphine elixir or methadone) on a time-contingent rather than as-needed basis may represent a beneficial adjunct to the pain relief provided by sympathetic neural blockade. Because many patients suffering from acute herpes zoster are elderly or may have severe multisystem disease, close monitoring for the potential side effects of potent narcotic analgesics (e.g., confusion or dizziness, which may cause a patient to fall) is warranted. Daily dietary fiber supplementation and milk of magnesia should be started along with opioid analgesics to prevent the side effect of constipation.

Adjuvant Analgesics

The anticonvulsant gabapentin represents a first-line treatment in the palliation of neuritic pain of acute herpes zoster involving the geniculate ganglion. Recent studies also suggest that gabapentin may also help prevent the development of postherpetic neuralgia. Treatment with gabapentin should begin early in the course of the disease, and this drug may be used concurrently with neural blockade, opioid analgesics, and other adjuvant analgesics including the antidepressant compounds if care is taken to avoid central nervous system side effects. Gabapentin is started at a bedtime dose of 300 mg and is titrated upward in 300-mg increments to a maximum dose of 3600 mg given in divided doses as side effects allow. Carbamazepine should be considered in patients suffering from severe neuritic pain who have failed to respond to nerve blocks and gabapentin. If this drug is used, rigid monitoring for hematologic parameters, especially in patients receiving chemotherapy or radiation therapy, is indicated. Phenytoin may also be beneficial to treat neuritic pain but should not be used in patients with lymphoma

because the drug may induce a pseudolymphoma-like state that is difficult to distinguish from the actual lymphoma itself.

Antidepressants may also be useful adjuncts in the initial treatment of the patient suffering from acute herpes zoster. On an acute basis, these drugs help alleviate the significant sleep disturbance that is commonly seen in this setting. In addition, the antidepressants may be valuable in helping ameliorate the neuritic component of the pain, which is treated less effectively with narcotic analgesics. After several weeks of treatment, the antidepressants may exert a mood-elevating effect that may be desirable in some patients. Care must be taken to observe closely for central nervous system side effects in this patient population. These drugs may cause urinary retention and constipation that may be mistakenly attributed to herpes zoster myelitis.

Antiviral Agents

A limited number of antiviral agents, including famciclovir and acyclovir, have been shown to shorten the course of acute herpes zoster and may help prevent the development of acute herpes zoster. They are probably useful in attenuating the disease in immunosuppressed patients. These antiviral agents can be used in conjunction with the treatment modalities mentioned earlier. Careful monitoring for side effects is mandatory with the use of these drugs.

Adjunctive Treatments

The application of ice packs to the lesions of acute herpes zoster may provide relief in some patients. Application of heat increases pain in most patients, presumably because of increased conduction of small fibers, but is beneficial in an occasional patient and may be worth trying if application of cold is ineffective. Transcutaneous electrical nerve stimulation and vibration may also be effective in a limited number of patients. The favorable risk-to-benefit ratio of all these modalities makes them reasonable alternatives for patients who cannot or will not undergo sympathetic neural blockade and tolerate pharmacologic interventions.

Topical application of aluminum sulfate as a tepid soak provides excellent drying of the crusting and weeping lesions of acute herpes zoster, and most patients find these soaks soothing. Zinc oxide ointment may also be used as a protective agent, especially during the healing phase when temperature sensitivity is a problem. Disposable diapers can be used as an absorbent padding to protect healing lesions from contact with clothing and sheets.

COMPLICATIONS

In most patients, acute herpes zoster involving the geniculate ganglion is a self-limited disease. In the elderly and the immunosuppressed, however, complications may occur. Cutaneous and visceral dissemination may range from a mild rash resembling chickenpox to an overwhelming, life-threatening infection in those already suffering from severe multisystem disease. Myelitis may cause bowel, bladder, and lower extremity paresis. Ocular complications from trigeminal nerve involvement may range from severe photophobia to keratitis with loss of sight.

CLINICAL PEARLS

Because the pain of herpes zoster usually precedes the eruption of skin lesions by 5 to 7 days, erroneous diagnosis of other painful conditions (e.g., trigeminal neuralgia, glaucoma) may be made. In this setting, the astute clinician will advise the patient to call immediately should rash appear as the diagnosis of acute herpes zoster is a possibility. Some pain specialists believe that in a small number of immunocompetent patients, when reactivation of virus occurs, a rapid immune response may attenuate the natural course of the disease and the characteristic rash of acute herpes zoster may not appear. This pain in the distribution of the geniculate ganglion without associated rash is called *zoster sine herpete* and is by necessity a diagnosis of exclusion. Therefore, other causes of head pain must first be ruled out before invoking this diagnosis.

Because of the potential for hearing loss in patients suffering from Ramsay Hunt syndrome, patients should be warned of this eventuality to avoid this complication being erroneously blamed on a therapeutic intervention, such as stellate ganglion block.

8 Eagle's Syndrome

ICD-9 CODE 756.71

THE CLINICAL SYNDROME

An uncommon cause of facial pain, Eagle's syndrome (also known as *stylohyoid syndrome*) is caused by pressure on the internal carotid artery and surrounding structures, including branches of the glossopharyngeal nerve, by an abnormally elongated styloid process and/or a calcified stylohyoid ligament. The pain of Eagle's syndrome is sharp and stabbing in nature and occurs with movement of the mandible or with turning of the neck. The pain starts below the angle of the mandible and radiates into the tonsillar fossa, temporomandibular joint, and base of the tongue. A trigger point may be present in the tonsillar fossa. Injection of the attachment of the stylohyoid ligament to the styloid process with local anesthetic and steroid will serve as both a diagnostic and therapeutic maneuver.

SIGNS AND SYMPTOMS

Eagle's syndrome is most often a diagnosis of exclusion. Patients suffering from Eagle's syndrome present with a history of sudden sharp, neuritic pain that begins below the angle of the mandible and radiates into the tonsillar fossa, temporomandibular joint, and base of the tongue. The pain is triggered by swallowing, movement of the mandible, or turning of the neck (Fig. 8–1). The intensity of pain is moderate to severe and unpleasant in character. On physical examination, the neurological examination is normal. The pain of Eagle's syndrome may be triggered by palpation of the tonsillar fossa.

TESTING

In patients suffering from Eagle's syndrome, radiographs and/or computed tomography scanning of the region of the styloid process demonstrate an elongated styloid process that is often associated with a calcified stylohyoid ligament. The diagnosis of Eagle's syndrome may be strengthened by a diagnostic injection of the attachment of the stylohyoid ligament to the styloid process with local anesthetic. Pain relief following this injection suggests a local etiology for the pain rather than a more distant cause, such as glossopharyngeal neuralgia or retropharyngeal tumor.

DIFFERENTIAL DIAGNOSIS

Eagle's syndrome can be distinguished from glossopharyngeal neuralgia in that the pain of glossopharyngeal neuralgia is characterized by paroxysms of shock-like pain in a manner analogous to trigeminal neuralgia rather than the sharp, shooting pain on movement that is associated with Eagle's syndrome. Because glossopharyngeal neuralgia may be associated with serious cardiac bradyarrhythmias and syncope, the clinician must distinguish the two syndromes.

The clinician should always evaluate the patient suffering from pain in this anatomic region for occult malignancy. Tumors of the larynx, hypopharynx, and anterior triangle of the neck may present with clinical symptoms identical to eagle's syndrome. Given the low incidence of Eagle's syndrome relative to pain secondary to malignancy in this anatomic region, Eagle's syndrome must be considered a diagnosis of exclusion.

TREATMENT

Many patient's suffering from Eagle's syndrome will respond to a series of therapeutic injections of the attachment of the stylohyoid ligament to the styloid process with local anesthetic and steroid. To perform this procedure, an imaginary line is visualized running from the mastoid process to the angle of the

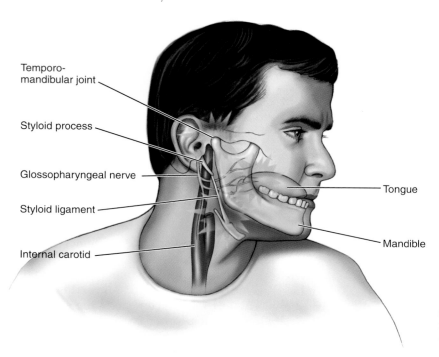

Temporo-
mandibular joint

Styloid process

Glossopharyngeal nerve

Styloid ligament

Internal carotid

Tongue

Mandible

Figure 8–1. The pain of Eagle's syndrome is triggered by swallowing, movement of the mandible, or turning of the neck.

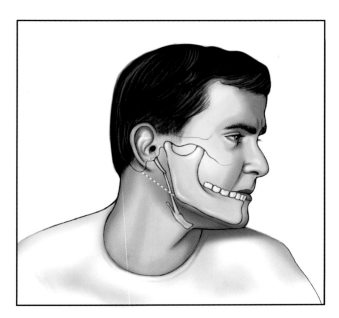

Figure 8–2. An imaginary line from the mastoid process to the angle of the mandible is an aid in needle placement for injection in a patient with Eagle's syndrome.

mandible (Fig. 8–2). The styloid process should lie just below the midpoint of this line. The skin is prepped with antiseptic solution. A 22-gauge × 1½-inch needle attached to a 10-mL syringe is advanced at this midpoint location in a plane perpendicular to the skin. The styloid process should be encountered within 3 cm. After contact is made, the needle is withdrawn slightly out of the periosteum or substance of the calcified ligament. After careful aspiration reveals no blood or cerebrospinal fluid, 5 mL of 0.5% preservative-free lidocaine combined with 80 mg of methylprednisolone is injected in incremental doses. Subsequent daily nerve blocks are carried out in a similar manner substituting 40 mg of methylprednisolone for the initial 80-mg dose.

The sharp shooting pain associated with Eagle's syndrome may also be treated with gabapentin. Gabapentin is started at a single nighttime dose of 300 mg and titrated upward by 300-mg increments every 2 days in divided doses until pain relief is achieved or a total daily dose of 3600 mg is reached. Alternatively, carbamazepine or phenytoin may be tried.

SIDE EFFECTS AND COMPLICATIONS

The major complications associated with this injection technique are related to trauma to the internal jugular and carotid artery. Hematoma formation and intravascular injection of local anesthetic with subsequent toxicity are not uncommon complications of this technique. Inadvertent blockade of the motor portion of the glossopharyngeal nerve can result in dysphagia secondary to weakness of the stylopharyngeus muscle. If the vagus nerve is inadvertently blocked, dysphonia secondary to paralysis of the ipsilateral vocal cord may occur. A reflex tachycardia secondary to vagal nerve block is also observed in some patients. Inadvertent block of the hypoglossal and spinal accessory nerves during glossopharyngeal nerve block will result in weakness of the tongue and trapezius muscle.

CLINICAL PEARLS

Eagle's syndrome is an uncommon cause of facial pain. Given the low incidence of Eagle's syndrome relative to pain secondary to malignancy in this anatomic region, Eagle's syndrome must be considered a diagnosis of exclusion. The clinician should always evaluate the patient suffering from pain in this anatomic region for occult malignancy. Tumors of the larynx, hypopharynx, and anterior triangle of the neck may present with clinical symptoms identical to Eagle's syndrome.

9 *Omohyoid Syndrome*

THE CLINICAL SYNDROME

Trauma is the common denominator in patients suffering from omohyoid syndrome. The syndrome is most often seen in patients who have recently suffered a bout of intense vomiting or sustained a flexion/extension injury to the cervical spine and to the musculature of the anterior neck. The pain of omohyoid syndrome is the result of damage to the fibers of the inferior belly of the omohyoid muscle. This pain presents as myofascial in nature. It is constant and exacerbated with movement of the affected muscle. A trigger point in the inferior belly of the omohyoid muscle is often present and provides a basis for treatment. The pain of omohyoid syndrome starts just above the clavicle at the lateral aspect of the clavicular attachment of the sternocleidomastoid muscle. The pain may radiate into the anterolateral neck. Injection of the trigger point in the inferior muscle of the omohyoid muscle with local anesthetic and steroid serves as both a diagnostic and therapeutic maneuver.

SIGNS AND SYMPTOMS

The patient suffering from omohyoid syndrome presents with pain in the supraclavicular region at a point just lateral and superior to where the sterno-cleidomastoid muscle attaches to the clavicle (Fig. 9–1). The pain often radiates into the anterolateral neck and increases with movement of the omohyoid muscle. There is a baseline level of pain even without movement of the muscle. The pain intensity ranges from minor to moderate. A trigger point in the belly of the omohyoid muscle is often present. The neurological examination of the patient suffering from

omohyoid syndrome is normal unless there has also been trauma to the cervical nerve roots or brachial plexus.

TESTING

Magnetic resonance imaging (MRI) of the soft tissues of the neck may reveal hematoma formation of the omohyoid muscle acutely and calcification and/or fibrosis as the syndrome becomes more chronic. Injection of the belly of the omohyoid muscle with local anesthetic can serve as a diagnostic maneuver to help strengthen the diagnosis.

DIFFERENTIAL DIAGNOSIS

Soft tissue injuries to the region may mimic omohyoid syndrome. Because trauma is invariably involved in the evolution of the painful condition, it is not surprising that the strain and sprain of other soft tissues often exist concurrently with omohyoid syndrome. Primary or metastatic tumors of the neck and hypopharynx may also mimic the clinical presentation of omohyoid syndrome and should be high on the list of diagnostic possibilities if the history of trauma is weak or absent.

TREATMENT

The nonsteroidal anti-inflammatory agents or cyclooxygenase-2 (COX-2) inhibitors represent a reasonable first step in the treatment of omohyoid syndrome. The use of the tricyclic antidepressants such as nortriptyline at a single bedtime dose of 25 mg titrating upward as side effects allow will also be useful, especially if sleep disturbance is also present. The injection of trigger points in the inferior belly of the omohyoid muscle often produces dramatic improvement in the patient's pain symptomatology.

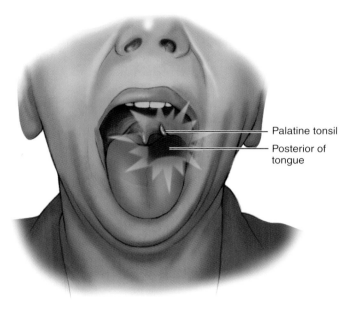

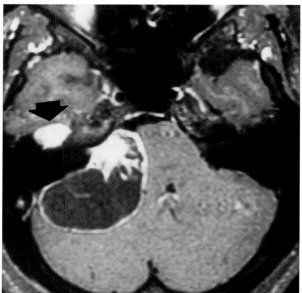

Palatine tonsil

Posterior of tongue

Figure 10–1. The pain of glossopharyngeal neuralgia is in the distribution of the ninth cranial nerve.

Figure 10–2. Mixed cystic and solid acoustic nerve schwannoma in association with a solid schwannoma of the geniculate ganglion. *A,* Axial enhanced image with fat saturation. There is a large mass in the right cerebellopontine angle (CPA) with solid and cystic enhancing components. There is a separate solid erosive tumor in the region of the right geniculate ganglion (*arrowhead*). *B,* Coronal enhanced image with fat saturation. The characteristic mushroom appearance of an intracanalicular acoustic schwannoma with extension into the adjacent CPA is well seen. This more anterior section through the internal auditory canal does not demonstrate the cystic portion of the tumor but nicely shows the compression of the adjacent brainstem. (From Stark DD, Bradley WG Jr [eds]: Magnetic Resonance Imaging, Vol III, 3rd ed. St Louis, Mosby, 1999, p. 1219.)

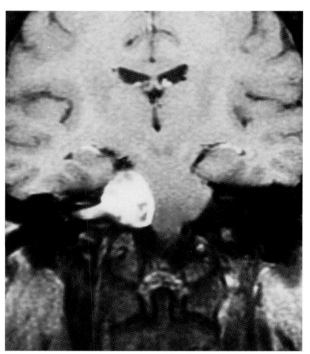

Diseases of the eye, ears, nose, throat, and teeth may all mimic trigeminal neuralgia or may coexist and confuse the diagnosis. Tumors of the hypopharynx including the tonsillar fossa and piriform sinus may mimic the pain of glossopharyngeal neuralgia, as will tumors at the cerebellopontine angle. Occasionally, demyelinating disease may produce a clinical syndrome identical to glossopharyngeal neuralgia. The jaw claudication associated with temporal arteritis also sometimes confuses the clinical picture, as may trigeminal neuralgia.

TREATMENT

Drug Therapy

Carbamazepine

This drug is considered first-line treatment for glossopharyngeal neuralgia. In fact, rapid response to this drug essentially confirms a clinical diagnosis of glossopharyngeal neuralgia. Despite the safety and efficacy of carbamazepine compared with other treatments for glossopharyngeal neuralgia, much confusion and unfounded anxiety surround its use. This medication, which may be the patient's best chance for pain control, is sometimes discontinued due to laboratory abnormalities erroneously attributed to it. Therefore, baseline screening laboratory tests, consisting of a complete blood cell count, urinalysis, and automated chemistry profile, should be obtained before starting the drug.

Carbamazepine should be started slowly if the pain is not out of control at a starting dose of 100 to 200 mg at bedtime for 2 nights, and the patient should be cautioned regarding side effects, including dizziness, sedation, confusion, and rash. The drug is increased in 100- to 200-mg increments, given in equally divided doses over 2 days, as side effects allow until pain relief is obtained or a total dose of 1200 mg daily is reached. Careful monitoring of laboratory parameters is mandatory to avoid the rare possibility of life-threatening blood dyscrasia. At the first sign of blood count abnormality or rash, this drug should be discontinued. Failure to monitor patients started on carbamazepine can be disastrous because aplastic anemia can occur. When pain relief is obtained, the patient should be kept at that dosage of carbamazepine for at least 6 months before considering tapering of this medication. The patient should be informed that under no circumstances should the dosage of drug be changed or the drug refilled or discontinued without the physician's knowledge.

Gabapentin

In the uncommon event that carbamazepine does not adequately control a patient's pain, gabapentin may be considered. As with carbamazepine, baseline blood tests should be obtained before starting therapy. Start with a 300-mg dose of gabapentin at bedtime for 2 nights, and caution the patient about potential side effects, including dizziness, sedation, confusion, and rash. The drug is then increased in 300-mg increments, given in equally divided doses over 2 days, as side effects allow until pain relief is obtained or a total dose of 2400 mg daily is reached. At this point, if the patient has experienced partial relief of pain, blood values are measured and the drug is carefully titrated upward using 100-mg tablets. Rarely will more than 3600 mg daily be required.

Baclofen

This drug has been reported to be of value in some patients who fail to obtain relief from the above-mentioned medications. Baseline laboratory tests should also be obtained before starting baclofen. Start with a 10-mg dose at bedtime for 2 nights, and caution the patient about potential adverse effects, which are the same as those of carbamazepine and gabapentin. The drug is increased in 10-mg increments, given in equally divided doses over 7 days as side effects allow, until pain relief is obtained or a total dose of 80 mg daily is reached. This drug has significant hepatic and central nervous system side effects, including weakness and sedation. As with carbamazepine, careful monitoring of laboratory values is indicated during the initial use of this drug.

In treating individuals with any of the drugs mentioned, the clinician should make the patient aware that premature tapering or discontinuation of the medication may lead to the recurrence of pain and that it will be more difficult to control pain thereafter.

Invasive Therapy

Glossopharyngeal Nerve Block

The use of glossopharyngeal nerve block with local anesthetic and a steroid serves as an excellent adjunct to drug treatment of glossopharyngeal neuralgia. This technique rapidly relieves pain while medications are being titrated to effective levels. The initial block is carried out with preservative-free bupivacaine combined with methylprednisolone. Subsequent daily nerve blocks are carried out in a similar manner substituting a lower dose of methylprednisolone. This approach may also be used to obtain control of breakthrough pain.

Radiofrequency Destruction of the Glossopharyngeal Nerve

The destruction of the glossopharyngeal nerve can be carried out by creating a radiofrequency lesion under biplanar fluoroscopic guidance. This procedure is reserved for patients who have failed to respond to all the treatments mentioned for intractable glossopharyngeal neuralgia and are not candidates for microvascular decompression of the glossopharyngeal root.

Microvascular Decompression of the Glossopharyngeal Root

This technique, which is also called *Janetta's procedure,* is the major neurosurgical procedure of choice for intractable glossopharyngeal neuralgia. It is based on the theory that glossopharyngeal neuralgia is in fact a compressive mononeuropathy. The operation consists of identifying the glossopharyngeal root close to the brainstem and isolating the offending compressing blood vessel. A sponge is then interposed between the vessel and nerve, relieving the compression and thus the pain.

CLINICAL PEARLS

The pain of glossopharyngeal neuralgia is among the most severe pain that mankind suffers from and thus must be considered a medical emergency. The uncontrolled pain of glossopharyngeal neuralgia has led to suicide, and strong consideration to the hospitalization of such patients should be given. Between attacks of glossopharyngeal neuralgia, the patient is relatively pain free. If a dull ache remains after the intense pain subsides, this is highly suggestive of a persistent compression of the nerve by a structural lesion such as a brainstem tumor or schwannoma. Glossopharyngeal neuralgia is almost never seen in people under 30 unless it is associated with multiple sclerosis, and all such patients should undergo MRI with sequences designed to identify demyelinating disease.

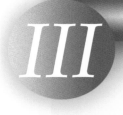

III

Neck and Brachial Plexus Pain Syndromes

11 *Spasmodic Torticollis*

ICD-9 CODE 333.83

THE CLINICAL SYNDROME

Spasmodic torticollis is a rare condition characterized by involuntary movement of the head. It is classified as a focal or segmental dystonia and occurs in approximately 3 in 10,000 people. It begins in early adult life. There are three varieties of spasmodic torticollis.

■ Tonic, which involves involuntary turning of the head to one side
■ Clonic, which involves involuntary shaking of the head
■ Tonic/clonic, which involves both types of involuntary movement

Spasmodic torticollis can also be subclassified as to the specific movement of the head: (1) rotation, which involves the turning of the head to the side; (2) laterocollis, which involves the leaning of the head against the shoulder; (3) retrocollis, which involves the leaning of the head toward the back; and (4) anterocollis, which involves the leaning of the head toward the chest. The disease occurs more commonly in women and is often initially diagnosed as a hysterical reaction or tic.

Thought to be due to dysfunction centrally, rather than a disease of the affected muscles, spasmodic torticollis often begins a subtle involuntary movement of the head. Early in the disease the dystonia is often intermittent. As the disease progresses, the symptoms become more severe and harder for the patient to hide. The dystonic movements may become more sustained and associated with constant, aching pain in the affected muscles. The pain often becomes the primary reason for the patient to seek medical attention, with the patient almost indifferent to the dystonic movements. The dystonia often disappears with sleep and becomes less pronounced on first awakening with the dystonic movements and pain worsening as the day progresses. Spontaneous recovery has been reported but overall, treatment is difficult and of limited success.

SIGNS AND SYMPTOMS

The patient suffering from spasmodic torticollis exhibits involuntary, dystonic movements of the head. In extreme cases, the dystonia will be continuous and the laterocollis so marked that the patient's ear will rest on the ipsilateral shoulder (Fig. 11–1). Pain may be a predominant feature of the syndrome, and spasms of the cervical paraspinous musculature, the strap muscles of the neck, and the sternocleidomastoid are often present. Hypertrophy of the affected muscles may occasionally occur. Other than the dystonic movements, the neurological examination is normal. As mentioned above, the patient may exhibit a seeming indifference to his or her abnormal head movements or position. Often, touching the opposite side of the face or chin will cause the dystonia to momentarily cease.

TESTING

Magnetic resonance imaging (MRI) of the brain and brainstem should be performed on all patients suspected of suffering from spasmodic torticollis. MRI of the brain provides the clinician with the best information regarding the cranial vault and its contents. MRI is highly accurate and helps to identify abnormalities that may put the patient at risk for neurological disasters due to intracranial and brainstem pathology, including tumors and demyelinating disease. Magnetic resonance angiography (MRA) may be useful to help identify aneurysms responsible for the patient's neurological symptomatology. In patients who cannot undergo MRI, such as a patient

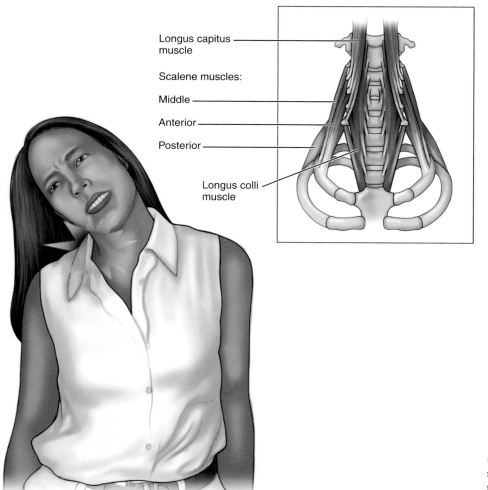

Longus capitus muscle

Scalene muscles:

Middle

Anterior

Posterior

Longus colli muscle

Figure 11–1. The dystonia of spasmodic torticollis causes significant pain and functional disability.

with a pacemaker, computed tomography (CT) scanning is a reasonable second choice.

Clinical laboratory testing consisting of a complete blood cell count, automated chemistry profile, and erythrocyte sedimentation rate are indicated to rule out infection and malignancy.

DIFFERENTIAL DIAGNOSIS

Spasmodic torticollis is generally a straightforward clinical diagnosis that can be made on the basis of a targeted history and physical examination. The involuntary nature of this movement disorder is the hallmark of the disease and helps distinguish it from tics and habit spasms that are voluntary and worsen when the patient is tense. Both tics and habit spasms resemble volitional movement. Behavioral abnormalities such as hysterical conversion reactions must also be considered. Acute spasm and pain of the muscles of the neck or wry neck can mimic spasmodic torticollis, but its onset is acute and the symptoms usually resolve within days to a week. Occasionally, patients with clonic spasmodic torticollis are initially diagnosed as having Parkinson's disease.

TREATMENT

In general, the treatment of spasmodic torticollis is disappointing. Pharmacological treatment with the skeletal muscle relaxants, drugs that act at the spinal cord level such as baclofen, and centrally acting drugs, including the anticonvulsants and L-dopa, may provide some symptomatic relief in mild cases. Trihexyphenidyl and diazepam have also been advocated.

For those patients for whom pharmacological treatment fails, injection of the affected muscles with botulinum toxin is a reasonable next step. Frequent injections may result in the development of antibodies against the toxin, which makes the toxin less effective. By changing to different subtypes of toxin, efficacy may be restored. For intractable cases, bilateral thalamotomy has been advocated. The results of this radical treatment are variable at best.

CLINICAL PEARLS

Spasmodic torticollis is a devastating disease that responds poorly to treatment. Injection of the affected muscles with botulinum toxin to effect chemodenervation is probably the best therapeutic option for most patients. The diagnosis of the disease is relatively straightforward. MRI of the bran is indicated in all patients thought to suffer from spasmodic torticollis.

12
Cervicothoracic Interspinous Bursitis

ICD-9 CODE 727.3

THE CLINICAL SYNDROME

Cervicothoracic interspinous bursitis is an uncommon cause of pain in the lower cervical and upper thoracic spine. The interspinous ligaments of the lower cervical and upper thoracic spine and their associated muscles are susceptible to the development of acute and chronic pain symptomatology following overuse. It is thought that bursitis is responsible for this pain syndrome. Frequently, the patient presents with midline pain after prolonged activity requiring hyperextension of the neck such as painting a ceiling or following the prolonged use of a computer monitor with too high of a focal point. The pain is localized to the interspinous region between C7 and T1 and does not radiate. It is constant, dull, and aching in character. The patient may attempt to relieve the constant ache by assuming a posture of dorsal kyphosis with a thrusting forward of the neck (Fig. 12–1). The pain of cervicothoracic interspinous bursitis often improves with activity and is made worse with rest and relaxation.

SIGNS AND SYMPTOMS

The patient suffering from cervicothoracic bursitis will present with the complaint of dull, poorly localized pain in the lower cervical and upper thoracic region. The pain spreads from the midline to the adjacent paraspinous area, but is nonradicular in nature. The patient often holds the cervical spine rigid with the head thrust forward to splint the affected ligament and bursae. Flexion and extension of the lower cervical spine and upper thoracic spine tend to cause more pain than rotation of the head.

The neurological examination of patients suffering from cervicothoracic bursitis should be normal. Focal or radicular neurological findings suggest a central or spinal cord origin of the patient's pain symptomatology and should be followed up with magnetic resonance imaging (MRI) of the appropriate anatomic regions.

TESTING

MRI of the lower cervical and upper thoracic spine should be carried out on all patients thought to be suffering from cervicothoracic bursitis. Electromyography of the brachial plexus and upper extremities is indicated if there are neurological findings or pain that radiates into the arms. Clinical laboratory testing consisting of a complete blood cell count, automated chemistry profile, antinuclear antibody testing, and erythrocyte sedimentation rate are indicated to rule out infection, collagen vascular disease including ankylosing spondylitis, and malignancy that may mimic the clinical presentation of cervicothoracic bursitis. Injection of the affected interspinous bursae with local anesthetic and steroid may serve as both a diagnostic and therapeutic maneuver and may help strengthen the diagnosis of cervicothoracic bursitis. Plain radiography of the sacroiliac joints is indicated if ankylosing spondylitis is being considered in the differential diagnosis.

DIFFERENTIAL DIAGNOSIS

The diagnosis of cervicothoracic bursitis is usually made on clinical grounds as a diagnosis of exclusion. The clinician needs to rule intrinsic disease of the spinal cord, including syringomyelia and tumor, which may mimic the clinical presentation of cervicothoracic bursitis. Ankylosing spondylitis may also present in a manner similar to that of cervicothoracic bursitis. Fibromyalgia may coexist with cervicotho-

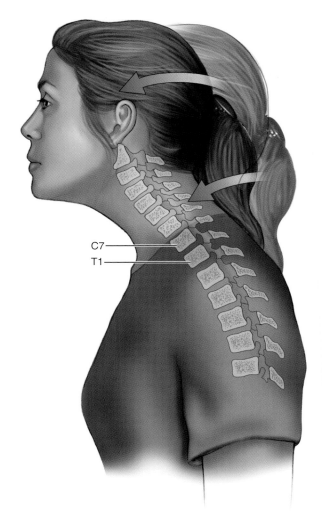

C7

T1

Figure 12–1. Patients suffering from cervicothoracic interspinous bursitis attempt to relieve their pain by assuming a position of dorsal kyphosis with a thrusting forward of the neck.

racic bursitis and should be identifiable by its characteristic trigger points and positive jump sign.

TREATMENT

Initial treatment of the pain and functional disability associated with cervicothoracic bursitis should include a combination of the nonsteroidal anti-inflammatory agents or cyclooxygenase-2 (COX-2) inhibitors and physical therapy. The local application of heat and cold may also be beneficial. For patients who do not respond to these treatment modalities, the following injection technique with a local anesthetic and steroid may be a reasonable next step.

The skin overlying the C7-T1 interspace is prepared with antiseptic solution. A syringe containing 3.0 mL of 0.25% preservative-free bupivacaine and

40 mg of methylprednisolone is attached to a 1½-inch 25-gauge needle. The needle is then carefully advanced through the supraspinal ligament into the interspinous ligament (Fig. 12–2). Care must be taken to keep the needle in the midline and not to advance it too deeply or inadvertent epidural, subdural, or subarachnoid injection could occur. After careful aspiration, a volume of 2 to 3 mL is then gently injected into the ligament. A series of two to five treatment sessions may be required to completely abolish the symptoms of cervicothoracic bursitis, and the patient should be informed of such.

SIDE EFFECTS AND COMPLICATIONS

The proximity to the spinal cord and exiting nerve roots makes it imperative that this procedure be carried out only by those well versed in the regional anatomy and experienced in performing injection techniques. The proximity to the vertebral artery combined with the vascular nature of this anatomic region makes the potential for intravascular injection high. Even small amounts of a local anesthetic injected into the vertebral arteries will result in seizures. Given the proximity of the brain and brainstem, ataxia following trigger point injection due to vascular uptake of local anesthetic is not an uncommon occurrence. Many patients will also complain of a transient increase in pain following injection in the above-mentioned anatomic area. If long needles are used, pneumothorax may also occur.

Because of the proximity of the epidural, subdural, and subarachnoid space, placement of a needle too deeply could result in inadvertent neuraxial block. Failure to recognize inadvertent epidural, subdural, or dural puncture can result in significant motor and sensory block with the potential for associated loss of consciousness, hypotension, and apnea. If subdural placement is unrecognized and the above doses of local anesthetics are administered, the signs and symptoms are similar to that of subarachnoid injection, although the resulting motor and sensory block may be spotty.

CLINICAL PEARLS

This injection technique is extremely effective in the treatment of cervicothoracic bursitis. This technique is a safe procedure if careful attention is paid to the clinically relevant anatomy in the areas to be injected. Care must be taken to use sterile technique to avoid infection as well as the use of universal precautions to avoid risk to the operator. Most side effects of the injection technique for cervicothoracic

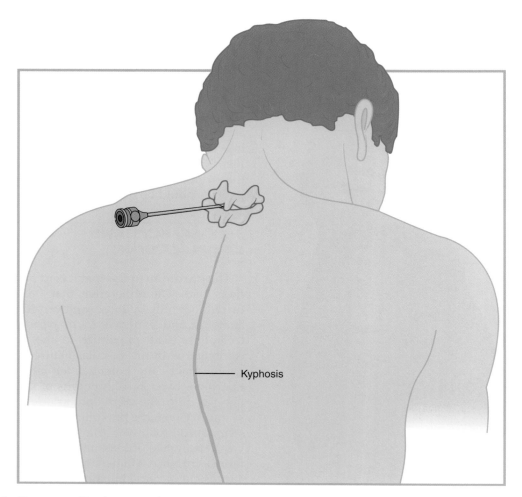

Kyphosis

Figure 12–2. Proper needle placement for injection for treatment of cervicothoracic interspinous bursitis pain. (From Waldman SD: Atlas of Pain Management Injection Techniques. Philadelphia, WB Saunders, 2000, p 33.)

bursitis are related to needle-induced trauma to the injection site and underlying tissues. The incidence of ecchymosis and hematoma formation can be decreased if pressure is placed on the injection site immediately after injection. The avoidance of overly long needles help decrease the incidence of trauma to underlying structures. Special care must be taken to avoid pneumothorax given the proximity to the underlying pleural space.

The use of physical modalities, including local heat as well as gentle stretching exercises, should be introduced several days after the patient undergoes this injection technique for cervicothoracic bursitis. Vigorous exercises should be avoided because they will exacerbate the patient's symptomatology. Simple analgesics, nonsteroidal anti-inflammatory agents, and antimyotonic agents such as tizanidine may be used concurrently with this injection technique.

13

Scapulocostal Syndrome

ICD-9 CODE 726.2

THE CLINICAL SYNDROME

Scapulocostal syndrome is a clinical syndrome characterized by pain and paresthesias over the medial border of the scapula that radiates into the neck, upper triceps, chest wall, and the distal upper extremity. The pain is burning and aching in nature. The intensity level of pain associated with scapulocostal syndrome is moderate.

Also known as *traveling salesman shoulder*, scapulocostal syndrome is thought to be an overuse syndrome due to repetitive use of the shoulder stabilizing muscles, including the serratus anterior, levator scapulae, pectoralis minor, and rhomboid, when carrying out activities such as reaching backward over a car seat for samples and prolonged use of the telephone cradled between the shoulder and neck (Fig. 13–1). Racquet sports have also been implicated in the evolution of scapulocostal syndrome.

SIGNS AND SYMPTOMS

Physical examination will reveal myofascial trigger points in the rhomboid, infraspinatus, and subscapularis muscles. These trigger points are best demonstrated by having the patient reach across the chest and place his or her hand on the uninvolved shoulder. Palpation of trigger points along the medial border of the scapula will produce a positive jump sign and cause pain to radiate into the ipsilateral upper extremity. The neurological examination of the upper extremity is normal in scapulocostal syndrome. Untreated, patients with scapulocostal syndrome will develop decreased range of motion of the shoulder and scapula, resulting in functional disability and pain.

TESTING

Plain radiographs are indicated in all patients who present with scapulocostal syndrome. Based on the patient's clinical presentation, additional testing including complete blood cell count, sedimentation rate, and antinuclear antibody testing may be indicated. Magnetic resonance imaging (MRI) of the shoulder is indicated if rotator cuff tear is suspected. Radionuclide bone scanning is indicated if metastatic disease or primary tumor involving the shoulder is being considered. Chest radiographs with apical lordotic views should be obtained if superior sulcus tumor of the lung is a possibility. Electromyography and nerve conduction velocity testing will help rule out radiculopathy, brachial plexopathy, and entrapment neuropathy.

DIFFERENTIAL DIAGNOSIS

Scapulocostal syndrome is most commonly misdiagnosed as cervical radiculopathy. However, in contradistinction to cervical radiculopathy, which is associated with numbness and weakness in the affected dermatomes, the upper extremity neurological examination in scapulocostal syndrome is normal. Osteoarthritis, rheumatoid arthritis, posttraumatic arthritis, and rotator cuff tear arthropathy are also common causes of shoulder pain secondary to arthritis that may be confused with scapulocostal syndrome. Less common causes of arthritis-induced shoulder pain include the collagen vascular diseases, infection, villonodular synovitis, and Lyme disease. Acute infectious arthritis is usually accompanied by significant systemic symptoms including fever and malaise and should be easily recognized by the astute clinician and treated appropriately with culture and antibiotics, rather than injection therapy. The collagen vascular diseases will generally present as a polyarthropathy rather than a monoarthropathy limited

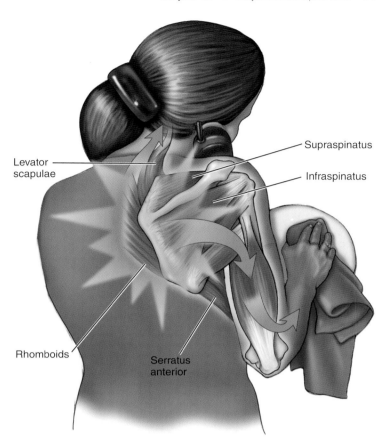

Figure 13–1. Scapulocostal syndrome is due to repetitive use of the shoulder stabilizing muscles.

to the shoulder joint, and the pain does not radiate into the upper extremity. Pancoast's tumor and brachial plexopathy may also mimic the clinical presentation of scapulocostal syndrome.

TREATMENT

Initial treatment of the pain and functional disability associated with scapulocostal syndrome should include a combination of the nonsteroidal anti-inflammatory agents or cyclooxygenase-2 (COX-2) inhibitors and physical therapy. The local application of heat and cold may also be beneficial. Avoidance of repetitive movements that incite the syndrome should be avoided. For patients who do not respond to these treatment modalities, injection of myofascial trigger points with local anesthetic and steroid may be a reasonable next step.

SIDE EFFECTS AND COMPLICATIONS

The major complication in the care of the patient suspected of suffering from scapulocostal syndrome is misdiagnosis. Tumors of the superior sulcus of the lung or primary or metastatic tumors of the shoulder and scapula must be included in the differential diagnosis.

CLINICAL PEARLS

Scapulocostal syndrome is a less common cause of shoulder and upper extremity pain encountered in clinical practice, with cervical radiculopathy occurring much more commonly. This painful condition must be separated from other causes of shoulder pain, including rotator cuff tears. Coexistent bursitis and tendinitis may also contribute to shoulder pain and may require additional treatment with more localized injection of local anesthetic and depot-steroid. Trigger point injections are a safe procedure if careful attention is paid to the clinically relevant anatomy in the areas to be injected. Care must be taken to use sterile technique to avoid infection as well as the use of universal precautions to avoid risk to the operator. The incidence of ecchymosis and hematoma formation can be decreased if pressure is placed on the injection site immediately after injection. The use of physical modalities, including local heat as well as gentle range of motion exercises, should be introduced several days after the patient undergoes trigger point injections for scapulocostal syndrome. Avoidance of activities responsible for the evolution of the disease must be considered or the syndrome will recur. Vigorous exercises should be avoided because they will exacerbate the patient's symptomatology. Simple analgesics and nonsteroidal anti-inflammatory agents or a COX-2 inhibitor may be used concurrently with this injection technique.

14

Parsonage-Turner Syndrome

ICD-9 353.0

THE CLINICAL SYNDROME

First identified as a distinct clinical entity in 1948, Parsonage and Turner described the painful condition of the shoulder and upper extremity that bears their name. The pain of Parsonage-Turner syndrome is of acute onset and is severe in intensity. The pain is burning in character and involves the shoulder and upper arm, preceding the onset of muscle weakness by hours to days (Fig. 14–1). Sleep disturbance is common, and weakness of the muscles of the shoulder and upper extremity, including the deltoid, infraspinatus, supraspinatus, and biceps, occurs as the syndrome progresses. In some patients, this weakness can be severe, progressing to complete flaccidity. A viral etiology of Parsonage-Turner syndrome has been advanced, as has the belief that this painful condition is an immunological disease. Neither theory has been proved.

SIGNS AND SYMPTOMS

Patients suffering from Parsonage-Turner syndrome will first complain of the sudden onset of pain that begins in the shoulder and radiates down the arm. The pain is severe in intensity and is followed by the development of weakness. On physical examination, the skin examination will be normal with no evidence of acute herpes zoster. Range of motion of the cervical spine will generally not affect the patient's pain or numbness in contradistinction to cervical radiculopathy.

Weakness of the muscles of the shoulder and upper extremity, including the deltoid, infraspinatus, supraspinatus, and biceps, increases as the syndrome progresses. Flaccidity of these muscles may occur.

Usually, more than one portion of the brachial plexus is affected, although isolated single nerve involvement can occur.

DIFFERENTIAL DIAGNOSIS

There are numerous causes of the brachial plexopathy. In common to all of them is the constellation of symptoms consisting of neurogenic pain and associated weakness that radiates into the supraclavicular region and upper extremity. More common causes of brachial plexopathy include compression of the plexus by cervical ribs or abnormal muscles (e.g., thoracic outlet syndrome), invasion of the plexus by tumor (e.g., Pancoast's syndrome), direct trauma to the plexus (e.g., stretch injuries and avulsions), inflammatory causes (e.g., Parsonage-Turner syndrome), and postradiation plexopathy. Cervical radiculopathy is a much more common cause of upper extremity pain and weakness relative to Parsonage-Turner syndrome. Table 14–1 helps differentiate these two painful conditions. In patients in whom Parsonage-Turner syndrome affects only an isolated nerve, the syndrome may be misdiagnosed as an entrapment neuropathy.

Electromyography is the cornerstone in sorting out the differential diagnosis in patients with the acute onset of shoulder and upper extremity pain.

Diseases of the cervical spinal cord, the bony cervical spine, and disc can mimic Parsonage-Turner syndrome. Appropriate testing, including magnetic resonance imaging (MRI) and electromyography, helps to sort out the myriad possibilities, but the clinician should also be aware that more than one pathological process may coexist and contribute to the patient's symptomatology. Syringomyelia, tumors of the cervical spinal cord, and tumors of the cervical nerve roots as they exit the spinal cord, such as schwannomas, can be of insidious onset and quite difficult to diagnose. Pancoast's tumor should be high on the list of diagnostic possibilities in all

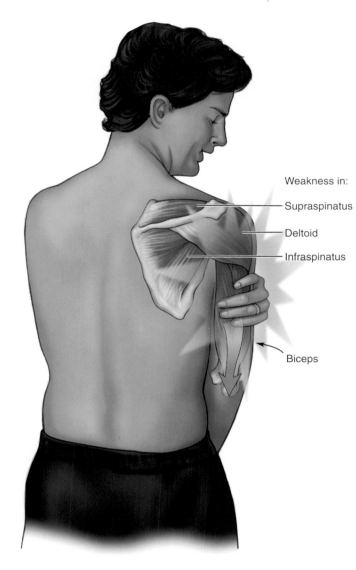

Weakness in:

Supraspinatus

Deltoid

Infraspinatus

Biceps

Figure 14–1. The pain of Parsonage-Turner syndrome involves the shoulder and upper arm, preceding the onset of muscle weakness by hours to days.

patients presenting with brachial plexopathy in the absence of clear antecedent trauma, especially if there is a past history of tobacco abuse. Lateral herniated cervical disc, metastatic tumor, or cervical spondylosis that results in significant nerve root compression may also present as a brachial plexopathy. Rarely, infection involving the apex of the lung may compress and irritate the plexus.

TESTING

All patients presenting with Parsonage-Turner syndrome must undergo MRI of the cervical spine

and the brachial plexus. Computed tomography (CT) scanning is a reasonable second choice if MRI is contraindicated. Electromyography and nerve conduction velocity testing are extremely sensitive, and the skilled electromyographer can help delineate the specific portion of the plexus that is abnormal. If an inflammatory basis for the plexopathy is suspected, serial electromyography is indicated. If Pancoast's tumor or other tumors of the brachial plexus are suspected, chest radiographs with apical lordotic views may be helpful. Screening laboratory testing consisting of complete blood cell count, erythrocyte sedimentation rate, antinuclear antibody testing, and automated blood chemistry testing should be performed if the diagnosis of brachial plexopathy is in question to help rule out other causes of the patient's pain.

TREATMENT

Drug Therapy

Gabapentin

Gabapentin is the first-line treatment for the neuritic pain of Parsonage-Turner syndrome. Start with a 300-mg dose of gabapentin at bedtime for 2 nights and caution the patient about potential side effects, including dizziness, sedation, confusion, and rash. The drug is then increased in 300-mg increments, given in equally divided doses over 2 days, as side effects allow until pain relief is obtained or a total dose of 2400 mg daily is reached. At this point, if the patient has experienced partial relief of pain, blood values are measured and the drug is carefully titrated upward using 100-mg tablets. Rarely will more than 3600 mg daily be required.

Carbamazepine

This drug is useful in those patients suffering from Parsonage-Turner syndrome who do not experience pain relief with gabapentin. Despite the safety and efficacy of carbamazepine compared with other treatments for Parsonage-Turner syndrome, much confusion and unfounded anxiety surrounds its use. This medication, which may be the patient's best chance for pain control, is sometimes discontinued due to laboratory abnormalities erroneously attributed to it. Therefore, baseline screening laboratory tests, consisting of a complete blood cell count, urinalysis, and automated chemistry profile, should be obtained before starting the drug.

Carbamazepine should be started slowly if the pain is not out of control. Start with a 100- to 200-mg dose at bedtime for 2 nights and caution the patient

Table 14–1. Comparison of Parsonage-Turner Syndrome with Cervical Radiculopathy

Syndrome	History	Examination	Test Results
Parsonage-Turner syndrome	Acute, intense burning pain that begins spontaneously in shoulder and upper arm; pain unaffected by neck movement	Neurological deficits that suggest more than one nerve is involved; weakness that may progress to flaccidity	Electromyogram positive for brachial plexopathy; magnetic resonance imaging of cervical spine noncontributory to diagnosis.
Cervical radiculopathy	Pain begins in neck and radiates down arm; the pain is increased by neck movement; pain and muscle weakness occur spontaneously	Weakness and numbness in the distribution of a single nerve root	Magnetic resonance imaging of cervical spine reveals herniated disc and/or osteophyte formation

regarding side effects, including dizziness, sedation, confusion, and rash. The drug is increased in 100- to 200-mg increments, given in equally divided doses over 2 days, as side effects allow until pain relief is obtained or a total dose of 1200 mg daily is reached. Careful monitoring of laboratory parameters is mandatory to avoid the rare possibility of life-threatening blood dyscrasia. At the first sign of blood count abnormality or rash, this drug should be discontinued. Failure to monitor patients started on carbamazepine can be disastrous because aplastic anemia can occur. When pain relief is obtained, the patient should be kept at that dosage of carbamazepine for at least 6 months before considering tapering of this medication. The patient should be informed that under no circumstances should the dosage of drug be changed or the drug refilled or discontinued without the physician's knowledge.

Baclofen

This drug has been reported to be of value in some patients who fail to obtain relief from the above-mentioned medications. Baseline laboratory tests should also be obtained before starting baclofen. Start with a 10-mg dose at bedtime for 2 nights and caution the patient about potential adverse effects, which are the same as those of carbamazepine and gabapentin. The drug is increased in 10-mg increments, given in equally divided doses over 7 days as side effects allow, until pain relief is obtained or a total dose of 80 mg daily is reached. This drug has significant hepatic and central nervous system side effects, including weakness and sedation. As with carbamazepine, careful monitoring of laboratory values is indicated during the initial use of this drug.

In treating individuals with any of the drugs mentioned, the physician should make the patient aware that premature tapering or discontinuation of the medication may lead to the recurrence of pain and that it will be more difficult to control pain thereafter.

Invasive Therapy

Brachial Plexus Block

The use of brachial plexus block with a local anesthetic and steroid serves as an excellent adjunct to drug treatment of Parsonage-Turner syndrome. This technique rapidly relieves pain while medications are being titrated to effective levels. The initial block is carried out with preservative-free bupivacaine combined with methylprednisolone. Subsequent daily nerve blocks are carried out in a similar manner substituting a lower dose of methylprednisolone. This approach may also be used to obtain control of breakthrough pain.

Physical Modalities

The use of physical and occupational therapy to maintain function and help palliate pain is a crucial part of the treatment plan for patients suffering from Parsonage-Turner syndrome. Shoulder abnormalities including subluxation and adhesive capsulitis must be aggressively searched for and treated. Occupation therapy to assist in activities of daily living is also important to avoid further deterioration of function.

COMPLICATIONS AND PITFALLS

The pain of Parsonage-Turner syndrome is difficult to treat. It responds poorly to opioid analgesics and may respond poorly to the above-mentioned medications.

The uncontrolled pain of Parsonage-Turner syndrome has led to suicide, and strong consideration to the hospitalization of such patients should be given. Correct diagnosis is crucial to successfully treat the pain and dysfunction associated with brachial plexopathy because stretch injuries and contusions of the plexus may respond with time, but plexopathy secondary to tumor or avulsion of the cervical roots will require aggressive treatment.

CLINICAL PEARLS

Brachial plexus block with a local anesthetic and steroid represents an excellent stop-gap measure for patients suffering from the uncontrolled pain of Parsonage-Turner syndrome while waiting for pharmacological treatments to take effect. As mentioned, correct diagnosis is paramount to allow the clinician to design a logical treatment plan for patients suffering from Parsonage-Turner syndrome.

15

Neck-Tongue Syndrome

ICD-9 CODE 729.2

THE CLINICAL SYNDROME

Neck-tongue syndrome is a rare condition characterized by pain in the neck associated with numbness of the ipsilateral half of the tongue that is aggravated by movement of the upper cervical spine. This unusual constellation of symptoms is thought to be due to compression of the C2 nerve root by compromise of the atlantoaxial joint. This compression can be caused by joint instability that allows subluxation of the lateral joint, bony abnormality such as congenital fusions or stenosis, or tubercular infection. The tongue numbness is thought to be due to damage or intermittent compression of the lingual afferent fibers that pass via the hypoglossal nerve to innervate the tongue. The bulk of the fibers are proprioceptive, and patients suffering from neck-tongue syndrome may also exhibit pseudoathetosis of the tongue. Neck-tongue syndrome occurs most commonly in patients older than 50 years, although the syndrome has been reported in a limited number of pediatric patients.

SIGNS AND SYMPTOMS

The pain of neck-tongue syndrome is in the distribution of the C2 nerve root. It is intermittent but is reproducible with certain neck movements. The physical findings associated with this pain are ill defined, with some patients suffering from neck-tongue syndrome exhibiting a decreased range of motion of the cervical spine or tenderness of the upper paraspinous musculature. The main objective finding in neck-tongue syndrome is the finding of decreased sensation of the ipsilateral half of the tongue (Fig. 15–1). Often associated with this finding

are pseudoathetoid movements of the tongue due to an impairment of the proprioceptive fibers.

TESTING

Magnetic resonance imaging (MRI) of the brain and brainstem should be performed on all patients suspected of suffering from neck-tongue syndrome. MRI of the brain provides the clinician with the best information regarding the cranial vault and its contents. MRI is highly accurate and helps to identify abnormalities that may put the patient at risk for neurological disasters due to intracranial and brainstem pathology, including tumors and demyelinating disease. Magnetic resonance angiography (MRA) may be useful to help identify aneurysms responsible for the patient's neurological symptomatology. In patients who cannot undergo MRI, such as a patient with a pacemaker, computed tomography (CT) is a reasonable second choice.

Clinical laboratory testing consisting of a complete blood cell count, automated chemistry profile, and erythrocyte sedimentation rate are indicated to rule out infection, temporal arteritis, and malignancy that may mimic neck-tongue syndrome. Endoscopy of the hypopharynx with special attention to the piriform sinuses is also indicated to rule out occult malignancy. Differential neural blockade of the C2 nerve may help strengthen the diagnosis of neck-tongue syndrome.

DIFFERENTIAL DIAGNOSIS

Neck-tongue syndrome is a clinical diagnosis that can be made of the basis of a targeted history and physical examination. Due to the rarity of this syndrome, the clinician must consider neck-tongue syndrome to be a diagnosis of exclusion. Diseases of the eye, ears, nose, throat, and teeth may coexist and confuse the diagnosis. Tumors of the hypopharynx,

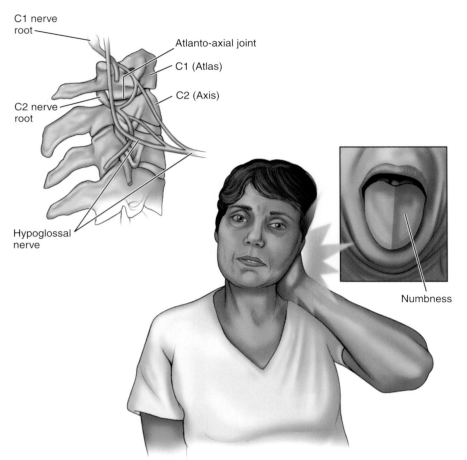

C1 nerve root

Atlanto-axial joint

C1 (Atlas)

C2 (Axis)

C2 nerve root

Hypoglossal nerve

Numbness

Figure 15–1. The pain and numbness of the ipsilateral half of the tongue are aggravated by movement of the upper cervical spine.

including the tonsillar fossa and piriform sinus, may mimic the pain of neck-tongue syndrome, as will tumors at the cerebellopontine angle. Occasionally, demyelinating disease may produce a clinical syndrome identical to neck-tongue syndrome. The jaw claudication associated with temporal arteritis may also sometimes confuse the clinical picture, as may glossopharyngeal neuralgia.

TREATMENT

The initial treatment of neck-tongue syndrome should consist of immobilization of the cervical spine with a soft cervical collar. A trial of the nonsteroidal anti-inflammatory agents or cyclooxygenase-2 (COX-2) inhibitors represents a reasonable next step. Block-ade of the atlantoaxial joint and C2 nerve root with a local anesthetic and steroid should also be considered. For refractory cases, cervical fusion of the upper cervical segments may be required.

CLINICAL PEARLS

Neck-tongue syndrome is a unique, but uncommon, cause of neck pain. The associated ipsilateral tongue numbness is pathognomonic for the syndrome and is unusual in character. An analogous type of proprioceptive numbness is seen in patients suffering from Bell's palsy. Given the rarity of this painful condition, the clinician should search carefully for other causes of the patient's symptomatology before attributing it to neck-tongue syndrome.

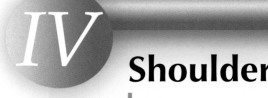

IV

Shoulder Pain Syndromes

16 *Suprascapular Nerve Entrapment*

THE CLINICAL SYNDROME

Suprascapular nerve entrapment is an uncommon cause of shoulder pain that is being encountered more frequently in clinical practice with the increasing use of backpacks instead of briefcases. Suprascapular nerve entrapment syndrome is caused by compression of the suprascapular nerve as it passes through the suprascapular notch. The most common causes of compression of the suprascapular nerve at this anatomic location include the prolonged wearing of heavy backpacks and direct blows to the nerve such as occur in football injuries and in falls from trampolines (Fig. 16–1). Suprascapular nerve entrapment syndrome is also seen in baseball pitchers and quarterbacks.

This entrapment neuropathy presents most commonly as a severe, deep, aching pain that radiates from the top of the scapula to the ipsilateral shoulder. Tenderness over the suprascapular notch is usually present. Shoulder movement, especially reaching across the chest, may increase the pain symptomatology. Untreated, weakness and atrophy of the supraspinatus and infraspinatus muscles will occur.

SIGNS AND SYMPTOMS

The most important finding in patients suffering from suprascapular nerve entrapment is weakness of the supraspinatus and infraspinatus muscles. This weakness manifests itself as weakness of abduction and external rotation of the ipsilateral shoulder. With significant compromise of the suprascapular nerve, atrophy of the infraspinatus muscle will be readily apparent as it lies superficially. The pain of suprascapular nerve entrapment can be exacerbated by abducting the ipsilateral scapula by reaching across the chest and simultaneously rotating the neck away from the involved shoulder. There often is tenderness to palpation of the suprascapular notch.

TESTING

Electromyography helps to distinguish cervical radiculopathy and Parsonage-Turner syndrome from suprascapular nerve entrapment syndrome. Plain radiographs are indicated in all patients who present with suprascapular nerve entrapment syndrome to rule out occult bony pathology. Based on the patient's clinical presentation, additional testing including complete blood cell count, uric acid, sedimentation rate, and antinuclear antibody testing may be indicated. Magnetic resonance imaging (MRI) of the shoulder is indicated if primary joint pathology or a space-occupying lesion is suspected. The injection technique described here serves as both a diagnostic and therapeutic maneuver.

DIFFERENTIAL DIAGNOSIS

Suprascapular nerve entrapment syndrome is often misdiagnosed as bursitis, tendinitis, or arthritis of the shoulder. Cervical radiculopathy of the C5 nerve root may also mimic the clinical presentation of suprascapular nerve entrapment syndrome. Parsonage-Turner syndrome, which is *idiopathic brachial neuritis,* may also present as sudden onset of shoulder pain and can be confused with suprascapular nerve entrapment. Tumor involving the superior scapular and/or shoulder should also be considered in the differential diagnosis of suprascapular nerve entrapment syndrome.

TREATMENT

The nonsteroidal anti-inflammatory agents or cyclooxygenase-2 (COX-2) inhibitors represent a

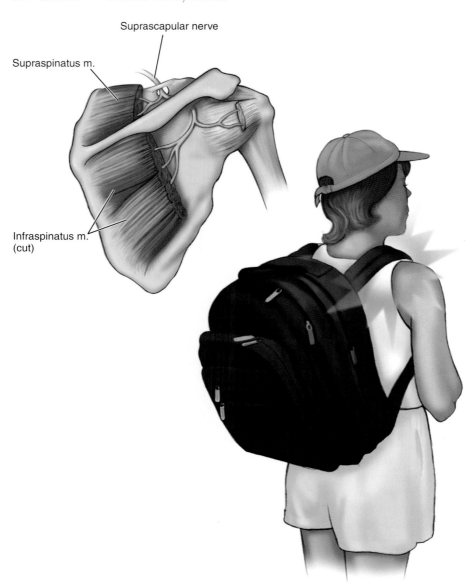

Suprascapular nerve

Supraspinatus m.

Infraspinatus m.
(cut)

Figure 16–1. Suprascapular nerve entrapment is caused by compression of the suprascapular nerve as it passes through the suprascapular notch.

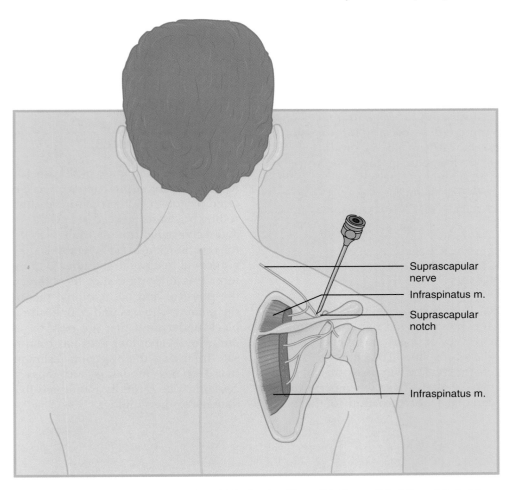

Suprascapular nerve

Infraspinatus m.

Suprascapular notch

Infraspinatus m.

Figure 16–2. Injection of suprascapular nerve for relief of pain. (From Waldman SD: Atlas of Pain Management Injection Techniques. Philadelphia, WB Saunders, 2000, p. 169.)

reasonable first step in the treatment of suprascapular nerve entrapment syndrome. The use of the tricyclic antidepressants such as nortriptyline at a single bedtime dose of 25 mg titrating upward as side effects allow will also be useful, especially if sleep disturbance is also present. Avoidance of repetitive trauma thought to be contributing to this entrapment neuropathy is also important, especially in professional athletes. If these maneuvers fail to produce rapid symptomatic relief, injection of the suprascapular nerve with local anesthetic and steroid is a reasonable next step (Fig. 16–2). If symptoms persist, surgical exploration and release of the suprascapular nerve are indicated.

SIDE EFFECTS AND COMPLICATIONS

The proximity to the suprascapular artery and vein suggests the potential for inadvertent intravascular injection and/or local anesthetic toxicity from intravascular absorption. The clinician should carefully calculate the total milligram dosage of local anesthetic that may be safely given when performing this injection technique. Due to proximity of the lung, should the needle be advanced too deeply through the suprascapular notch, pneumothorax is a possibility. Care must be taken if surgical decompression of the suprascapular nerve is undertaken to avoid inadvertent trauma to the spinal accessory nerve as it runs along the ventral surface of the trapezius.

CLINICAL PEARLS

Avoidance techniques of the repetitive movements responsible for suprascapular nerve entrapment are often forgotten in the rush to treatment. The use of rolling briefcases instead of backpacks may also help avoid continued trauma to the nerve. It is important for the clinician to be aware that this injection technique will render the shoulder joint insensate. Therefore, it is important that the clinician be sure that the physical and occupational therapists caring for the patient who has undergone suprascapular nerve block understand that not only the shoulder girdle but also the shoulder joint has been rendered insensate following this injection technique. This means that deep heat modalities and range of motion exercises must be carefully monitored to avoid burns or damage to the shoulder.

17 *Supraspinatus Tendinitis*

ICD-9 CODE 726.10

THE CLINICAL SYNDROME

Supraspinatus tendinitis can present as either an acute or a chronic painful condition of the shoulder. Acute supraspinatus tendinitis will usually occur in a younger group of patients following overuse or misuse of the shoulder joint. Inciting factors may include carrying heavy loads in front of and away from the body, throwing injuries, or the vigorous use of exercise equipment. Chronic supraspinatus tendinitis tends to occur in an older group of patients and to present in a more gradual or insidious manner without a single specific event of antecedent trauma. The pain of supraspinatus tendinitis will be constant and severe, with sleep disturbance often reported. The pain of supraspinatus tendinitis is felt primarily in the deltoid region. It is moderate to severe in intensity and may be associated with a gradual loss of range of motion of the affected shoulder. The patient often awakens at night when he or she rolls over onto the affected shoulder.

SIGNS AND SYMPTOMS

The patient suffering from supraspinatus tendinitis may attempt to splint the inflamed tendon by elevating the scapula to remove tension from the ligament, giving the patient a "shrugging" appearance (Fig. 17–1). There usually is point tenderness over the greater tuberosity. The patient will exhibit a painful arc of abduction, with the patient complaining of a catch or sudden onset of pain in the midrange of the arc due to impingement of the humeral head onto the supraspinatus tendon. Patients with supraspinatus tendinitis will exhibit a positive Dawbarn's sign, which is pain to palpation over the greater tuberosity of the humerus when the arm is

hanging down that disappears when the arm is fully abducted. Early in the course of the disease, passive range of motion is full and without pain. As the disease progresses, patients suffering from supraspinatus tendinitis often experience a gradual decrease in functional ability with decreasing shoulder range of motion, making simple everyday tasks such as hair combing, fastening a brassiere, or reaching overhead quite difficult. With continued disuse, muscle wasting may occur and a frozen shoulder may develop.

TESTING

Plain radiographs are indicated in all patients who present with shoulder pain. Based on the patient's clinical presentation, additional testing including complete blood cell count, sedimentation rate, and antinuclear antibody testing may be indicated. Magnetic resonance imaging (MRI) of the shoulder is indicated if rotator cuff tear is suspected (Fig. 17–2). The injection technique given here serves as both a diagnostic and therapeutic maneuver.

DIFFERENTIAL DIAGNOSIS

Because supraspinatus tendinitis may occur after seemingly minor trauma or develop gradually over time, the diagnosis often is delayed. Tendinitis of the musculotendinous unit of the shoulder frequently coexists with bursitis of the associated bursae of the shoulder joint, creating additional pain and functional disability. This ongoing pain and functional disability can cause the patient to splint the shoulder group with resultant abnormal movement of the shoulder, which puts additional stress on the rotator cuff. This can lead to further trauma to the entire rotator cuff. It should be remembered that with rotator cuff tears, passive range of motion is normal but active range of motion is limited, in contradistinction to frozen shoulder, where both passive and

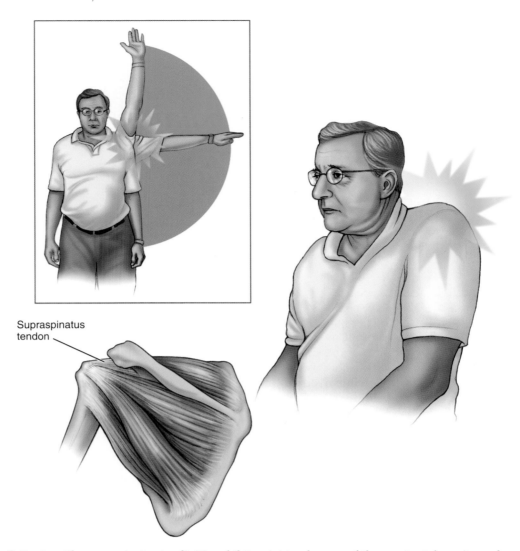

Supraspinatus
tendon

Figure 17–1. Patients with supraspinatus tendinitis exhibit point tenderness of the greater tuberosity and a painful arc of abduction.

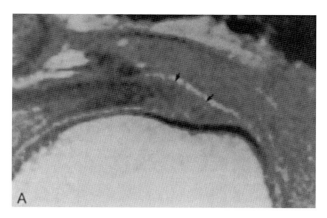

Figure 17–2. Tendinosis or tendinopathy of the rotator cuff. A coronal oblique protein density–weighted (TR/TE, 2000/25) spin-echo magnetic resonance image reveals increased signal intensity in the distal part of the supraspinatus tendon (*arrows*). There was no further increase in signal intensity in T2-weighted spin-echo magnetic resonance images. The peribursal fat plane is intact. (From Kjellin I, Ho CP, Cervilla V, et al: Alterations in the supraspinatus tendon at MR imaging: correlation with histopathologic findings in cadavers. Radiology 1991;181:837–841.)

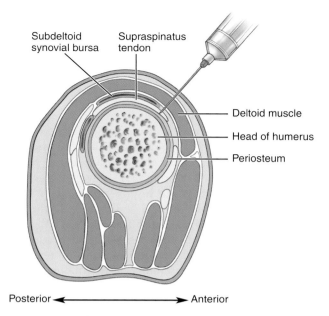

Figure 17–3. Correct needle placement for injection into the supraspinatus tendon.

active range of motion are limited. Rotator cuff tear rarely occurs before the age of 40 except in cases of severe acute trauma to the shoulder. Cervical radiculopathy may rarely cause pain limited to the shoulder, although in most instances, there is associated neck and upper extremity pain and numbness.

TREATMENT

Initial treatment of the pain and functional disability associated with supraspinatis tendinitis should include a combination of the nonsteroidal anti-inflammatory agents or cyclooxygenase-2 (COX-2) inhibitors and physical therapy. The local application of heat and cold may also be beneficial. For patients who do not respond to these treatment modalities, the following injection technique may be a reasonable next step. The use of physical therapy, including gentle range of motion exercises, should be introduced several days after the patient undergoes this injection technique for shoulder pain. Vigorous exercises should be avoided as they will exacerbate the patient's symptomatology.

To inject the supraspinatus tendon, the patient is placed in the supine position with the forearm medially rotated behind the back. This positioning of the upper extremity places the lateral epicondyle of the elbow in an anterior position and makes its identification easier. After identification of the lateral

epicondyle of the elbow, the humerus is traced superiorly to the anterior edge of the acromion. A slight indentation just below the anterior edge of the acromion marks the point of insertion of the supraspinatus tendon into the upper facet of the greater tuberosity of the humerus. The point is marked with a sterile marker.

Proper preparation with antiseptic solution of the skin overlying the shoulder, subacromial region, and joint space is then carried out. A sterile syringe containing 1.0 mL of 0.25% preservative-free bupivacaine and 40 mg of methylprednisolone is attached to a 25-gauge 1½-inch needle using strict aseptic technique. With strict aseptic technique, the previously marked point is palpated and the indentation indicating the insertion of the supraspinatus tendon is reidentified with the gloved finger. The needle is then carefully advanced perpendicularly at this point through the skin and subcutaneous tissues and through the joint capsule until it impinges on bone (Fig. 17–3). The needle is then withdrawn 1 to 2 mm out of the periosteum of the humerus, and the contents of the syringe are gently injected. There should be slight resistance to injection. If no resistance is encountered, either the needle tip is in the joint space itself or the supraspinatus tendon is ruptured. If there is significant resistance to injection, the needle tip is probably in the substance of a ligament or tendon and should be advanced or withdrawn slightly until the injection proceeds without significant resistance. The needle is then removed, and a sterile pressure dressing and ice pack are placed at the injection site.

SIDE EFFECTS AND COMPLICATIONS

The major complication of this injection technique is infection. This complication should be exceedingly rare if strict aseptic technique is adhered to. The possibility of trauma to the supraspinatus tendon from the injection itself remains an ever-present possibility. Tendons that are highly inflamed or previously damaged are subject to rupture if they are directly injected. This complication can be greatly decreased if the clinician uses gentle technique and stops injecting immediately if significant resistance to injection is encountered. Approximately 25% of patients will complain of a transient increase in pain following this injection technique and should be warned of such.

CLINICAL PEARLS

The musculotendinous unit of the shoulder joint is susceptible to the development of tendinitis for several reasons. First, the joint is subjected to a wide range of motions that are often repetitive in nature.

Second, the space in which the musculotendinous unit functions is restricted by the coracoacromial arch, making impingement a likely possibility with extreme movements of the joint. Third, the blood supply to the musculotendinous unit is poor, making healing of microtrauma more difficult. All of these factors can contribute to tendinitis of one or more of the tendons of the shoulder joint. Calcium deposition around the tendon may occur if the inflammation continues, making subsequent treatment more difficult. Tendinitis of the musculotendinous unit of the shoulder frequently coexists with bursitis of the associated bursae of the shoulder joint, creating additional pain and functional disability.

The injection technique described is extremely effective in the treatment of pain secondary to the causes of shoulder pain mentioned earlier. Coexistent bursitis and arthritis may also contribute to shoulder pain and may require additional treatment with a more localized injection of local anesthetic and depot steroid. This technique is a safe procedure if careful attention is paid to the clinically relevant anatomy in the areas to be injected. Care must be taken to utilize sterile technique to avoid infection as well as the use of universal precautions to avoid risk to the operator. The incidence of ecchymosis and hematoma formation can be decreased if pressure is placed on the injection site immediately following injection.

18

Infraspinatus Tendinitis

ICD-9 CODE 726.10

THE CLINICAL SYNDROME

Infraspinatus tendinitis can present as either an acute or a chronic painful condition of the shoulder. Acute infraspinatus tendinitis usually occurs in a younger group of patients after overuse or misuse of the shoulder joint. Inciting factors may include activities that require repeated abduction and lateral rotation of the humerus such as installing brake pads during assembly line work. The vigorous use of exercise equipment has also been implicated. The pain of infraspinatus tendinitis is constant and severe and is localized to the deltoid area. Significant sleep disturbance is often reported. Patients with infraspinatus tendinitis will exhibit pain with lateral rotation of the humerus and on active abduction. Chronic infraspinatus tendinitis tends to occur in an older group of patients and to present in a more gradual or insidious manner without a single specific event of antecedent trauma. The pain of infraspinatus tendinitis may be associated with a gradual loss of range of motion of the affected shoulder. The patient will often awaken at night when he or she rolls over onto the affected shoulder.

SIGNS AND SYMPTOMS

The patient may attempt to splint the inflamed infraspinatus tendon by rotating the scapula anteriorly to remove tension from the tendon (Fig. 18–1). There usually is point tenderness over the greater tuberosity. The patient will exhibit a painful arc of abduction, with the patient complaining of a catch or sudden onset of pain in the mid-range of the arc. Early in the course of the disease, passive range of motion is full and without pain. As the disease progresses, patients suffering from infraspinatus

tendinitis will often experience a gradual decrease in functional ability with decreasing shoulder range of motion, making simple everyday tasks such as hair combing, fastening a brassiere, or reaching overhead quite difficult. With continued disuse, muscle wasting may occur and a frozen shoulder may develop.

TESTING

Plain radiographs are indicated in all patients who present with shoulder pain. Based on the patient's clinical presentation, additional testing including complete blood cell count, sedimentation rate, and antinuclear antibody testing may be indicated. Magnetic resonance imaging (MRI) of the shoulder is indicated if rotator cuff tear is suspected. The injection technique given here serves as both a diagnostic and therapeutic maneuver.

DIFFERENTIAL DIAGNOSIS

Because infraspinatus tendinitis may occur after seemingly minor trauma or develop gradually over time, the diagnosis is often delayed. Tendinitis of the musculotendinous unit of the shoulder frequently coexists with bursitis of the associated bursae of the shoulder joint, creating additional pain and functional disability. This ongoing pain and functional disability can cause the patient to splint the shoulder group with resultant abnormal movement of the shoulder, which puts additional stress on the rotator cuff. This can lead to further trauma to the entire rotator cuff. It should be remembered that with rotator cuff tears, passive range of motion is normal, but active range of motion is limited, in contradistinction to frozen shoulder, where both passive and active range of motion are limited. Rotator cuff tear rarely occurs before the age of 40 except in cases of severe acute trauma to the shoulder. Cervical

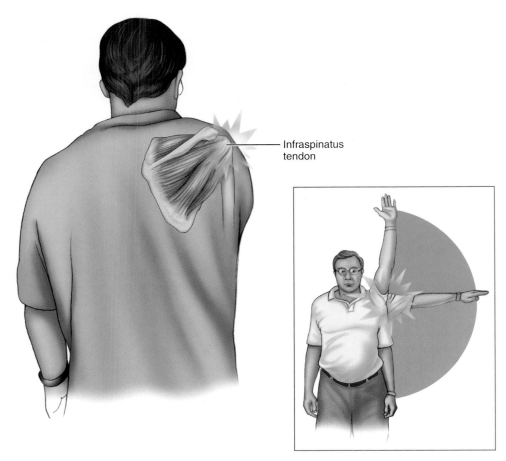

Infraspinatus
tendon

Figure 18–1. Patients suffering from infraspinatus tendinitis exhibit posterior point tenderness and a painful arc of abduction.

radiculopathy may rarely cause pain limited to the shoulder, although in most instances, there is associated neck and upper extremity pain and numbness.

TREATMENT

Initial treatment of the pain and functional disability associated with rotator cuff tear should include a combination of the nonsteroidal anti-inflammatory agents or cyclooxygenase-2 (COX-2) inhibitors and physical therapy. The local application of heat and cold may also be beneficial. For patients who do not respond to these treatment modalities, the following injection technique may be a reasonable next step. The use of physical therapy, including gentle range of motion exercises, should be introduced several days after the patient undergoes this injection technique for shoulder pain. Vigorous exercises should be avoided because they will exacerbate the patient's symptomatology.

To inject the infraspinatus tendon, the skin overlying the posterior shoulder is prepped with antiseptic solution. A sterile syringe containing 1.0 mL of 0.25% preservative-free bupivacaine and 40 mg of methylprednisolone is attached to a 25-gauge 1½-inch needle using strict aseptic technique. With strict aseptic technique, the previously marked point is palpated and the insertion of the infraspinatus tendon is reidentified with the gloved finger. The needle is then carefully advanced at this point through the skin and subcutaneous tissues as well as the margin of the deltoid muscle and underlying infraspinatus muscle until it impinges on bone (Fig. 18–2). The needle is then withdrawn 1 to 2 mm out of the periosteum of the humerus, and the contents of the syringe are gently injected. There should be slight resistance to injection. If no resistance is encountered, either the needle tip is in the joint space itself or the infraspinatus tendon is ruptured. If there is significant resistance to injection, the needle tip is probably in the substance of a ligament or tendon and should be advanced or withdrawn slightly until the injection proceeds without significant resistance. The needle is then removed, and a sterile pressure dressing and ice pack are placed at the injection site.

SIDE EFFECTS AND COMPLICATIONS

The major complication of this injection technique is infection. This complication should be exceedingly rare if strict aseptic technique is adhered to. The possibility of trauma to the infraspinatus tendon from the injection itself remains an ever-present possibil-

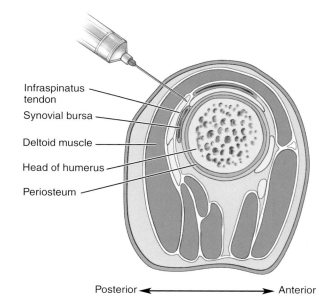

Figure 18–2. Correct needle placement for injection into the infraspinatus tendon.

ity. Tendons that are highly inflamed or previously damaged are subject to rupture if they are directly injected. This complication can be greatly decreased if the clinician uses gentle technique and stops injecting immediately if significant resistance to injection is encountered. Approximately 25% of patients will complain of a transient increase in pain after this injection technique and should be warned of such.

CLINICAL PEARLS

The musculotendinous unit of the shoulder joint is susceptible to the development of tendinitis for several reasons. First, the joint is subjected to a wide range of motions that are often repetitive in nature. Second, the space in which the musculotendinous unit functions is restricted by the coracoacromial arch, making impingement a likely possibility with extreme movements of the joint. Third, the blood supply to the musculotendinous unit is poor, making healing of microtrauma more difficult. All of these factors can contribute to tendinitis of one or more of the tendons of the shoulder joint. Calcium deposition around the tendon may occur if the inflammation continues, making subsequent treatment more difficult. Tendinitis of the musculotendinous unit of the shoulder frequently coexists with bursitis of the associated bursae of the shoulder joint, creating additional pain and functional disability.

The injection technique described is extremely effective in the treatment of pain secondary to the causes of shoulder pain mentioned. Coexistent bursitis and arthritis may also contribute to shoulder pain and may require additional treatment with a more localized injection of a local anesthetic and depot steroid. This technique is a safe procedure if careful attention is paid to the clinically relevant anatomy in the areas to be injected. Care must be taken to use sterile technique to avoid infection, as well as the use of universal precautions to avoid risk to the operator. The incidence of ecchymosis and hematoma formation can be decreased if pressure is placed on the injection site immediately after injection.

V

Elbow Pain Syndromes

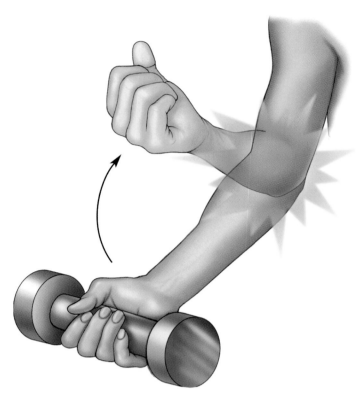

Figure 20–1. A patient suffering from cubital bursitis complains of pain and swelling on any movement of the elbow.

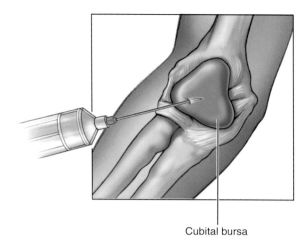

Cubital bursa

Figure 20–2. Proper needle placement for injection for treatment of cubital bursitis.

combination of the nonsteroidal anti-inflammatory agents or cyclooxygenase-2 (COX-2) inhibitors and physical therapy. The local application of heat and cold may also be beneficial. The repetitive movements that incite the syndrome should be avoided. For patients who do not respond to these treatment modalities, injection of the cubital bursa with a local anesthetic and steroid may be a reasonable next step (Fig. 20–2).

To inject the cubital bursa, the patient is placed in a supine position with the arm fully adducted at the patient's side and the elbow extended with the dorsum of the hand resting on a folded towel. A total of 2 mL of local anesthetic and 40 mg of methylprednisolone is drawn up in a 5-mL sterile syringe.

After sterile preparation of skin overlying the anterior aspect of the joint, the clinician then identifies the pulsations of the brachial artery at the crease of the elbow. After preparation of the skin with antiseptic solution, a 25-gauge 1-inch needle is inserted just lateral to the brachial artery at the crease and slowly advanced in a slightly medial and cephalic trajectory through the skin and subcutaneous tissues. If bone is encountered, the needle is withdrawn back into the subcutaneous tissue. The contents of the syringe are then gently injected. There should be little resistance to injection. If resistance is encountered, the needle is probably in the tendon and should be withdrawn back until the injection proceeds without significant resistance. The needle is then removed, and a sterile pressure dressing and ice pack are placed at the injection site.

SIDE EFFECTS AND COMPLICATIONS

The major complication associated with cubital diagnosis is misdiagnosis. Failure of the clinician to recognize an acute inflammatory or infectious arthritis of the elbow may result in permanent damage to the joint as well as chronic pain and functional disability. Injection of the cubital bursa at the elbow is a relatively safe block, with the major complications being inadvertent intravascular injection and persistent paresthesia secondary to needle trauma to the median nerve. This technique can be safely performed in the presence of anticoagulation by using a 25- or 27-gauge needle, albeit at increased risk of hematoma, if the clinical situation dictates a favorable risk-to-benefit ratio. These complications can be decreased if manual pressure is applied to the area of the block immediately after injection. Application of cold packs for 20-minute periods after the block will also decrease the amount of postprocedure pain and bleeding the patient may experience.

CLINICAL PEARLS

Bursae are formed from synovial sacs whose purpose it is to allow easy sliding of muscles and tendons across one another at areas of repeated movement. These synovial sacs are lined with a synovial membrane that is invested with a network of blood vessels that secrete synovial fluid. Inflammation of the bursa results in an increase in the production of synovial fluid with swelling of the bursal sac. With overuse or misuse, these bursae may become inflamed, enlarged, and, on rare occasions, infected. Coexistent tendinitis and epicondylitis may also contribute to elbow pain and may require additional treatment with more localized injection of local anesthetic and depot steroid. This technique is a safe procedure if careful attention is paid to the clinically relevant anatomy in the areas to be injected, in particular avoiding the median nerve by keeping the needle lateral to the brachial artery. Care must be taken to use sterile technique to avoid infection, as well as the use of universal precautions to avoid risk to the operator. The incidence of ecchymosis and hematoma formation can be decreased if pressure is placed on the injection site immediately after injection. The use of physical modalities, including local heat as well as gentle range of motion exercises, should be introduced several days after the patient undergoes this injection technique for elbow pain. Vigorous exercises should be avoided because they will exacerbate the patient's symptomatology. Simple analgesics and nonsteroidal anti-inflammatory agents may be used concurrently with this injection technique.

21 *Radial Tunnel Syndrome*

ICD-9 CODE 354.9

THE CLINICAL SYNDROME

Radial tunnel syndrome is an uncommon cause of lateral elbow pain that has the unique distinction among the entrapment neuropathies of almost always being initially misdiagnosed. The incidence of misdiagnosis of radial tunnel syndrome is in fact so common that it is often incorrectly referred to under the name of *resistant tennis elbow*. As will be seen from the following discussion, the only major similarity that radial tunnel syndrome and tennis elbow share is the fact that both clinical syndromes produce lateral elbow pain.

The lateral elbow pain of radial tunnel syndrome is aching in nature and is localized to the deep extensor muscle mass. The pain may radiate proximally and distally into the upper arm and forearm (Fig. 21–1). The intensity of the pain of radial tunnel syndrome is mild to moderate but may produce significant functional disability.

In radial tunnel syndrome, the posterior interosseous branch of the radial nerve is entrapped by a variety of mechanisms that have in common a similar clinical presentation. These mechanisms include aberrant fibrous bands in front of the radial head, anomalous blood vessels that compress the nerve, and/or a sharp tendinous margin of the extensor carpi radialis brevis. These entrapments may exist alone or in combination.

SIGNS AND SYMPTOMS

Regardless of the mechanism of entrapment of the radial nerve, the common clinical feature of radial tunnel syndrome is pain just below the lateral epicondyle of the humerus. The pain of radial tunnel syndrome may develop after an acute twisting injury or direct trauma to the soft tissues overlying the posterior interosseous branch of the radial nerve, or the onset may be more insidious without an obvious inciting factor. The pain is constant and is made worse with active supination of the wrist. Patients will often note the inability to hold a coffee cup or hammer. Sleep disturbance is common. On physical examination, elbow range of motion will be normal. Grip strength on the affected side may be diminished.

In the classic text on entrapment neuropathies, Dawson et al (Entrapment Neuropathies, 2nd ed. Little, Brown, 1990) note three important signs that will allow the clinician to distinguish radial tunnel syndrome from tennis elbow: (1) tenderness to palpation distal to the radial head in the muscle mass of the extensors rather than over the more proximal lateral epicondyle, as in tennis elbow; (2) increasing pain on active resisted supination of the forearm due to compression of the radial nerve by the arcade of Frohse as a result of contraction of the muscle mass; and (3) a positive result on the middle finger test. The middle finger test is performed by having the patient extend his or her forearm, wrist, and middle finger and sustain this action against resistance (Fig. 21–2). Patients suffering from radial tunnel syndrome will exhibit increased lateral elbow pain due to fixation and compression of the radial nerve by the extensor carpi radialis brevis muscle.

TESTING

Because of the ambiguity and confusion surrounding this clinical syndrome, testing is important to help confirm the diagnosis of radial tunnel syndrome. Electromyography helps to distinguish cervical radiculopathy and radial tunnel syndrome from tennis elbow. Plain radiographs are indicated in all patients who present with radial tunnel syndrome to rule out occult bony pathology. Based on the patient's clinical presentation, additional testing including complete blood cell count, uric acid, sedimentation rate, and

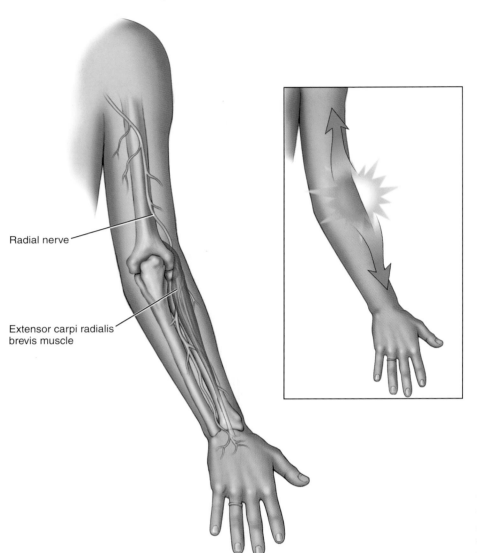

Radial nerve

Extensor carpi radialis
brevis muscle

Figure 21–1. The pain of radial
tunnel syndrome is localized to
the deep extensor muscle mass
and may radiate proximally and
distally into the upper arm and
forearm.

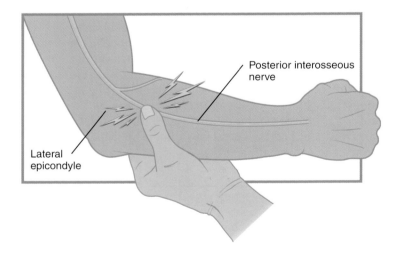

Posterior interosseous
nerve

Lateral
epicondyle

Figure 21–2. Radial tunnel syndrome can be
distinguished from tennis elbow by carefully
identifying the point of maximal tenderness.
(From Waldman SD: Atlas of Pain Management
Injection Techniques. Philadelphia, WB Saunders,
2000, p. 85.)

antinuclear antibody testing may be indicated. Magnetic resonance imaging (MRI) of the elbow is indicated if internal derangement of the joint is suspected and may also help identify the factors responsible for the nerve entrapment, such as ganglion cysts, lipomas, etc. The injection technique of the radial nerve at the elbow with a local anesthetic and steroid may help confirm the diagnosis as well as treat the syndrome.

DIFFERENTIAL DIAGNOSIS

Cervical radiculopathy and tennis elbow can mimic radial tunnel syndrome. Radial tunnel syndrome can be distinguished from tennis elbow in that with radial tunnel syndrome, the maximal tenderness to palpation is distal to the lateral epicondyle over the posterior interosseous branch of the radial nerve, whereas with tennis elbow, the maximal tenderness to palpation is over the lateral epicondyle. Increased pain with active supination as well as a positive middle finger test (see earlier) will help strengthen the diagnosis of radial tunnel syndrome. Acute gout affecting the elbow will present as a diffuse acute inflammatory condition that may be difficult to distinguish from infection of the joint, rather than a localized nerve entrapment.

TREATMENT

Initial treatment of the pain and functional disability associated with radial tunnel syndrome should include a combination of the nonsteroidal anti-inflammatory agents or cyclooxygenase-2 (COX-2) inhibitors and physical therapy. The local application of heat and cold may also be beneficial. The repetitive movements that incite the syndrome should be avoided. For patients who do not respond to these treatment modalities, injection of the radial nerve at the elbow with a local anesthetic and steroid may be a reasonable next step. If the symptoms of radial tunnel syndrome persist, surgical exploration and decompression of the radial nerve are indicated.

SIDE EFFECTS AND COMPLICATIONS

The major complications associated with radial tunnel syndrome fall into two categories: (1) iatrogenically induced complications due to persistent and overaggressive treatment of "resistant tennis elbow" and (2) the potential for permanent neurological deficits due to prolonged untreated entrapment of the radial nerve. Failure of the clinician to recognize an acute inflammatory or infectious arthritis of the elbow may result in permanent damage to the joint as well as chronic pain and functional disability.

CLINICAL PEARLS

Radial tunnel syndrome is a distinct clinical entity that is often misdiagnosed as tennis elbow, and this fact accounts for the many patients whose "tennis elbow" fails to respond to conservative measures. Radial tunnel syndrome can be distinguished from tennis elbow in that with radial tunnel syndrome, the maximal tenderness to palpation is over the radial nerve, whereas with tennis elbow, the maximal tenderness to palpation is over the lateral epicondyle. If radial tunnel syndrome is suspected, injection of the radial nerve at the humerus with a local anesthetic and steroid will give almost instantaneous relief. Careful neurological examination to identify preexisting neurological deficits that may later be attributed to the nerve block should be performed on all patients before beginning radial nerve block at the humerus.

22 *Anterior Interosseous Syndrome*

ICD-9 CODE 354.9

THE CLINICAL SYNDROME

Anterior interosseous syndrome is an uncommon cause of forearm and wrist pain. The onset of symptoms in patients suffering from anterior interosseous syndrome is usually after acute trauma to the forearm or after repetitive forearm and elbow motions such as using an ice pick. It is thought that in this setting, the pain and muscle weakness of anterior interosseous syndrome are secondary to median nerve compression of the nerve just below the elbow by the tendinous origins of the pronator teres muscle and flexor digitorum superficialis muscle of the long finger or by aberrant blood vessels. In some patients, no antecedent trauma is identified and an inflammatory etiology analogous to Parsonage-Turner syndrome has been suggested as the etiology of anterior interosseous syndrome in the absence of trauma.

Clinically, anterior interosseous syndrome presents as an acute pain in the proximal forearm and deep in the wrist. As the syndrome progresses, patients with anterior interosseous syndrome may complain about a tired or heavy sensation in the forearm with minimal activity as well as the inability to pinch items between the thumb and index finger due to paralysis of the flexor pollicis longis and the flexor digitorum profundus (Fig. 22–1).

SIGNS AND SYMPTOMS

Physical findings include the inability to flex the interphalangeal joint of the thumb and the distal interphalangeal joint of the index finger due to paralysis of the flexor pollicis longus and the flexor digitorum profundus. Tenderness over the forearm in the region of the pronator teres muscle is seen in some patients suffering from anterior interosseous syndrome. A positive Tinel's sign over the anterior interosseous branch of the median nerve approximately 6 to 8 cm below the elbow may also be present.

TESTING

Electromyography helps to distinguish cervical radiculopathy, thoracic outlet syndrome, and carpal tunnel syndrome from anterior interosseous syndrome. Plain radiographs are indicated in all patients who present with anterior interosseous syndrome to rule out occult bony pathology. Based on the patient's clinical presentation, additional testing including complete blood cell count, uric acid, sedimentation rate, and antinuclear antibody testing may be indicated. Magnetic resonance imaging (MRI) of the forearm is indicated if primary elbow pathology or a space-occupying lesion is suspected. The injection of the median nerve at the elbow will serve as both a diagnostic and therapeutic maneuver.

DIFFERENTIAL DIAGNOSIS

The anterior interosseous syndrome should also be differentiated from cervical radiculopathy involving the C6 or C7 roots that may at times mimic median nerve compression. Furthermore, it should be remembered that cervical radiculopathy and median nerve entrapment may coexist as the "double crush" syndrome. The double crush syndrome is seen most commonly with median nerve entrapment at the wrist or carpal tunnel syndrome. Anterior interosseous syndrome can be distinguished from pronator syndrome and median nerve compression by the ligament of Struthers in that the pain of anterior interosseous syndrome occurs more distally and is accompanied by the characteristic loss of ability to pinch items between the thumb and index finger.

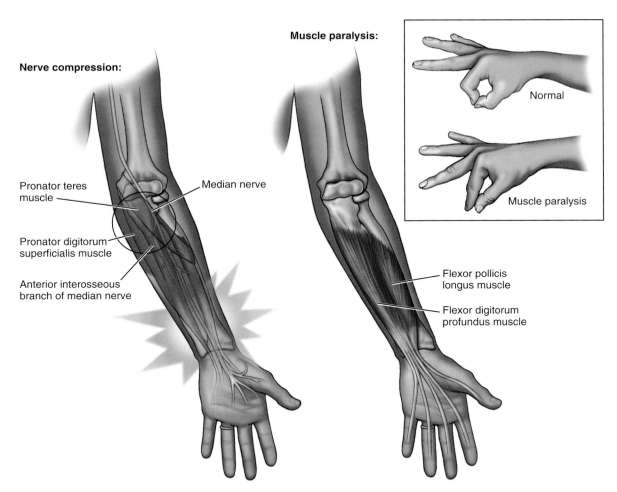

Nerve compression:

Pronator teres muscle

Pronator digitorum superficialis muscle

Anterior interosseous branch of median nerve

Median nerve

Muscle paralysis:

Flexor pollicis longus muscle

Flexor digitorum profundus muscle

Normal

Muscle paralysis

Figure 22–1. Patients suffering from anterior interosseous syndrome exhibit acute forearm pain and progressive weakness of pinch.

TREATMENT

The nonsteroidal anti-inflammatory agents or cyclooxygenase-2 (COX-2) inhibitors represent a reasonable first step in the treatment of anterior interosseous syndrome. The use of the tricyclic antidepressants such as nortriptyline at a single bedtime dose of 25 mg titrating upward as side effects allow will also be useful, especially if sleep disturbance is also present. Avoidance of repetitive trauma thought to be contributing to this entrapment neuropathy is also important. If these maneuvers fail to produce rapid symptomatic relief, injection of the median nerve at the elbow with a local anesthetic and steroid is a reasonable next step. If symptoms continue to persist, surgical exploration and release of the anterior interosseous branch of the median nerve are indicated.

SIDE EFFECTS AND COMPLICATIONS

Median nerve block below the elbow is a relatively safe block, with the major complications being inadvertent intravascular injection and persistent paresthesia secondary to needle trauma to the nerve. This technique can safely be performed in the presence of anticoagulation by using a 25- or 27-gauge needle, albeit at increased risk of hematoma, if the clinical situation dictates a favorable risk-to-benefit ratio. These complications can be decreased if manual pressure is applied to the area of the block immediately after injection. Application of cold packs for 20-minute periods after the block will also decrease the amount of postprocedure pain and bleeding the patient may experience.

CLINICAL PEARLS

Avoidance techniques of the repetitive movements responsible for pronator syndrome are often forgotten in the rush to treatment. Median nerve block at the elbow is a simple and safe technique in the evaluation and treatment of the afore-mentioned painful conditions. Careful neurological examination to identify preexisting neurological deficits that may later be attributed to the nerve block should be performed on all patients before beginning median nerve block at the elbow.

23 *Cubital Tunnel Syndrome*

ICD-9 CODE 354.2

THE CLINICAL SYNDROME

Cubital tunnel syndrome is an uncommon cause of lateral forearm pain and weakness that can be quite distressing to the patient. This entrapment neuropathy presents as pain and associated paresthesias in the lateral forearm that radiates to the wrist and ring and little fingers. The symptoms are often aggravated by prolonged flexion of the elbow. The pain of cubital tunnel syndrome has been characterized as unpleasant and dysesthetic. The onset of symptoms is usually after repetitive elbow motions or from repeated pressure on the elbow such as using the elbows to arise from bed. Direct trauma to the ulnar nerve as it enters the cubital tunnel may also result in a similar clinical presentation. Untreated, progressive motor deficit and, ultimately, flexion contracture of the affected fingers can result. Cubital tunnel syndrome is most often caused by compression of the ulnar nerve by an aponeurotic band that runs from the medial epicondyle of the humerus to the medial border of the olecranon.

SIGNS AND SYMPTOMS

Physical findings include tenderness over the ulnar nerve at the elbow. A positive Tinel's sign over the ulnar nerve as it passes beneath the aponeuroses is usually present. Weakness of the intrinsic muscles of the forearm and hand that are innervated by the ulnar nerve may be identified with careful manual muscle testing, although early in the course of the evolution of cubital tunnel syndrome, the only physical finding other than tenderness over the nerve may be the loss of sensation on the ulnar side of the little finger. As the syndrome progresses, the affected hand may take on a claw-like appearance (Fig. 23–1). A positive Wartenberg's sign indicative of weakness of the adduction of the fifth digit is often present.

TESTING

Electromyography helps to distinguish cervical radiculopathy and cubital tunnel syndrome from golfer's elbow. Plain radiographs are indicated in all patients who present with cubital tunnel syndrome to rule out occult bony pathology, such as osteophytes impinging on the ulnar nerve. Based on the patient's clinical presentation, additional testing including complete blood cell count, uric acid, sedimentation rate, and antinuclear antibody testing may be indicated. Magnetic resonance imaging (MRI) of the elbow is indicated if joint instability is suspected. Injection of the ulnar nerve will serve as both a diagnostic and therapeutic maneuver.

DIFFERENTIAL DIAGNOSIS

Cubital tunnel syndrome is often misdiagnosed as golfer's elbow, and this fact accounts for the many patients whose "golfer's elbow" fails to respond to conservative measures. Cubital tunnel syndrome can be distinguished from golfer's elbow in that in cubital tunnel syndrome, the maximal tenderness to palpation is over the ulnar nerve 1 inch below the medial epicondyle, whereas with golfer's elbow, the maximal tenderness to palpation is directly over the medial epicondyle. Cubital tunnel syndrome should also be differentiated from cervical radiculopathy involving the C7 or C8 roots and golfer's elbow. Furthermore, it should be remembered that cervical radiculopathy and ulnar nerve entrapment may coexist as the "double crush" syndrome. The double crush syndrome is seen most commonly with median nerve entrapment at the wrist or carpal tunnel syndrome.

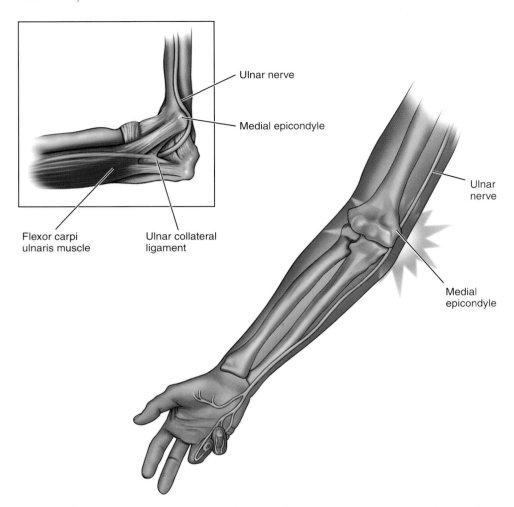

Figure 23–1. Patients suffering from cubital tunnel syndrome exhibit weakness of the intrinsic muscles of the forearm, and the hand may take on a "claw-like" appearance.

TREATMENT

Initial treatment of the pain and functional disability associated with cubital tunnel syndrome should include a combination of the nonsteroidal anti-inflammatory agents or cyclooxygenase-2 (COX-2) inhibitors and physical therapy. The local application of heat and cold may also be beneficial. The repetitive movements that incite the syndrome should be avoided. For patients who do not respond to these treatment modalities, injection of the ulnar nerve at the elbow with a local anesthetic and steroid may be a reasonable next step. If the symptoms of cubital tunnel syndrome persist, surgical exploration and decompression of the ulnar nerve are indicated.

SIDE EFFECTS AND COMPLICATIONS

The major complications associated with cubital tunnel syndrome fall into two categories: (1) iatrogenically induced complications due to persistent and overaggressive treatment of "resistant golfer's elbow" and (2) the potential for permanent neurological deficits due to prolonged untreated entrapment of the ulnar nerve. Failure of the clinician to recognize an acute inflammatory or infectious arthritis of the elbow may result in permanent damage to the joint as well as chronic pain and functional disability.

CLINICAL PEARLS

Cubital tunnel syndrome is a distinct clinical entity that is often misdiagnosed as golfer's elbow, and this fact accounts for the many patients whose "golfer's elbow" fails to respond to conservative measures. Cubital tunnel syndrome can be distinguished from golfer's elbow in that with cubital tunnel syndrome, the maximal tenderness to palpation is over the ulnar nerve and a positive Tinel's sign is present, whereas with golfer's elbow, the maximal tenderness to palpation is over the medial epicondyle. If cubital tunnel syndrome is suspected, injection of the radial nerve at the elbow with a local anesthetic and steroid will give almost instantaneous relief. Careful neurological examination to identify preexisting neurological deficits that may later be attributed to the nerve block should be performed on all patients before beginning ulnar nerve block at the elbow.

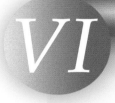

VI

Wrist and Hand
Pain Syndromes

24 Ulnar Tunnel Syndrome

ICD-9 CODE 354.2

THE CLINICAL SYNDROME

Ulnar tunnel syndrome is an entrapment neuropathy of the ulnar nerve that is characterized by pain numbness, and paresthesias of the wrist that radiate into the ulnar aspect of the palm and dorsum of the hand and the little finger as well as the ulnar half of the ring finger (Fig. 24–1). These symptoms may also radiate proximal to the nerve entrapment into the forearm. The pain of ulnar tunnel syndrome is often described as aching or burning in nature with associated "pins and needles"–like paresthesias.

Like carpal tunnel syndrome, ulnar tunnel syndrome occurs more commonly in women than in men. Also like carpal tunnel syndrome, the pain of ulnar tunnel syndrome is frequently worse at night and made worse by vigorous flexion and extension of the wrist. The onset of symptoms is usually after repetitive wrist motions or from direct trauma to the wrist such as wrist fractures or direct trauma to the proximal hypothenar eminence that may occur when the hand is used to hammer on hubcaps or from handlebar compression during long-distance cycling. Ulnar tunnel syndrome is also seen in patients with rapid weight gain, rheumatoid arthritis, or Dupuytren's disease or during pregnancy. Untreated, progressive motor deficit and, ultimately, flexion contracture of the affected fingers can result.

Ulnar tunnel syndrome is caused by compression of the ulnar nerve as it passes through Guyon's canal at the wrist. The most common causes of compression of the ulnar nerve at this anatomical location include space-occupying lesions including ganglion cysts and ulnar artery aneurysms, fractures of the distal ulna and carpals, and repetitive motion injuries that compromise the ulnar nerve as it passes though this closed space. This entrapment neuropathy presents most commonly as a pure motor neuropathy without pain, which is due to compression of the deep palmar branch of the ulnar nerve as it passes through Guyon's canal. This pure motor neuropathy presents as painless paralysis of the intrinsic muscles of the hand. Ulnar tunnel syndrome may also present as a mixed sensory and motor neuropathy. Clinically, this mixed neuropathy presents as pain as well as the motor deficits described above.

SIGNS AND SYMPTOMS

Physical findings include tenderness over the ulnar nerve at the wrist. A positive Tinel's sign over the ulnar nerve as it passes beneath the transverse carpal ligament is usually present. If the sensory branches are involved, there will be decreased sensation into the ulnar aspect of the hand and the little finger as well as the ulnar half of the ring finger. Depending on the location of neural compromise, the patient may have weakness of the intrinsic muscles of the hand as evidenced by the inability to spread the fingers and/or weakness of the hypothenar eminence.

TESTING

Electromyography helps to distinguish cervical radiculopathy, diabetic polyneuropathy, and Pancoast's tumor from ulnar tunnel syndrome. Plain radiographs are indicated in all patients who present with ulnar tunnel syndrome to rule out occult bony pathology. Based on the patient's clinical presentation, additional testing including complete blood cell count, uric acid, sedimentation rate, and antinuclear antibody testing may be indicated. Magnetic resonance imaging (MRI) of the wrist is indicated if joint instability or a space-occupying lesion is suspected. The injection technique described here will serve as both a diagnostic and therapeutic maneuver.

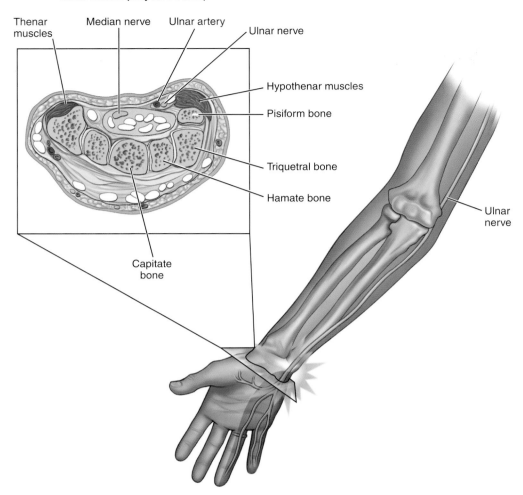

Figure 24–1. Ulnar tunnel syndrome is characterized by lateral forearm pain and weakness.

DIFFERENTIAL DIAGNOSIS

Ulnar tunnel syndrome is often misdiagnosed as arthritis of the carpometacarpal joints, cervical radiculopathy, Pancoast's tumor, and diabetic neuropathy. Patients with arthritis of the carpometacarpal joint will usually have radiographic evidence and physical findings suggestive of arthritis. Most patients suffering from a cervical radiculopathy will have reflex, motor, and sensory changes associated with neck pain, whereas patients with ulnar tunnel syndrome will have no reflex changes and motor and sensory changes will be limited to the distal ulnar nerve. Diabetic polyneuropathy generally presents as symmetrical sensory deficit involving the entire hand rather than limited just in the distribution of the ulnar nerve. It should be remembered that cervical radiculopathy and ulnar nerve entrapment may coexist as the "double crush" syndrome. Furthermore, because ulnar tunnel syndrome is commonly seen in patients with diabetes, it is not surprising that diabetic polyneuropathy usually presents in diabetic patients with ulnar tunnel syndrome. Pancoast's tumor invading the medial cord of the brachial plexus may also mimic an isolated ulnar nerve entrapment and should be ruled out by apical lordotic chest radiographs.

TREATMENT

Initial treatment of the pain and functional disability associated with ulnar tunnel syndrome should include a combination of the nonsteroidal anti-inflammatory agents or cyclooxygenase-2 (COX-2) inhibitors and physical therapy. The local application of heat and cold may also be beneficial. The repetitive movements that incite the syndrome should be avoided. For patients who do not respond to these treatment modalities, injection of the ulnar nerve at the ulnar tunnel with a local anesthetic and steroid may be a reasonable next step. If the symptoms of ulnar tunnel syndrome persist, surgical exploration and decompression of the ulnar nerve are indicated.

SIDE EFFECTS AND COMPLICATIONS

The major complication associated with ulnar tunnel syndrome is due to delayed diagnosis and treatment of the disease. This can result in permanent neurological deficits due to prolonged untreated entrapment of the ulnar nerve. Failure of the clinician to recognize an acute inflammatory or infectious arthritis of the wrist may result in permanent damage to the joint as well as chronic pain and functional disability.

CLINICAL PEARLS

Ulnar tunnel syndrome should also be differentiated from cervical radiculopathy involving the C8 spinal root that may at times mimic ulnar nerve compression. Furthermore, it should be remembered that cervical radiculopathy and ulnar nerve entrapment may coexist in the "double crush" syndrome. The double crush syndrome is seen most commonly with ulnar nerve entrapment at the wrist or carpal tunnel syndrome. Pancoast's tumor invading the medial cord of the brachial plexus may also mimic an isolated ulnar nerve entrapment and should be ruled out by apical lordotic chest radiographs.

25 Cheiralgia Paresthetica

THE CLINICAL SYNDROME

Cheiralgia paresthetica is an uncommon cause of wrist and hand pain and numbness. It is also known as *handcuff neuropathy*. The onset of symptoms of cheiralgia paresthetica is usually after compression of the sensory branch of the radial nerve. Radial nerve dysfunction secondary to compression by tight handcuffs, wristwatch bands, or casts is a common cause of cheiralgia paresthetica.

Direct trauma to the nerve may also result in a similar clinical presentation. Fractures or lacerations frequently completely disrupt the nerve, resulting in sensory deficit in the distribution of the radial nerve. The sensory branch of the radial nerve may also be damaged during surgical treatment of de Quervain's tenosynovitis.

Cheiralgia paresthetica presents as pain and associated paresthesias and numbness of the radial aspect of the dorsum of the hand to the base of the thumb (Fig. 25–1). Because there is significant interpatient variability in the distribution of the sensory branch of the radial nerve due to overlap of the lateral antebrachial cutaneous nerve, the signs and symptoms of cheiralgia paresthetica may vary from patient to patient.

SIGNS AND SYMPTOMS

Physical findings include tenderness over the radial nerve at the wrist. A positive Tinel's sign over the radial nerve at the distal forearm is usually present. Decreased sensation in the distribution of the sensory branch of the radial nerve is often present, although as mentioned, the overlap of the lateral antebrachial cutaneous nerve may result in a confusing clinical presentation. Flexion and pronation of the wrist as well as ulnar deviation often cause paresthesias in the distribution of the sensory branch of the radial nerve in patients suffering from cheiralgia paresthetica.

TESTING

Electromyography can help to identify the exact source of neurological dysfunction and to clarify the differential diagnosis and thus should be the starting point of the evaluation of all patients suspected of having cheiralgia paresthetica. Plain radiographs are indicated in all patients who present with cheiralgia paresthetica to rule out occult bony pathology. Based on the patient's clinical presentation, additional testing including complete blood cell count, uric acid, sedimentation rate, and antinuclear antibody testing may be indicated. Magnetic resonance imaging (MRI) of the elbow is indicated if joint instability is suspected. Injection of the sensory branch of the radial nerve at the wrist will serve as both a diagnostic and therapeutic maneuver and may be used as an anatomical differential neural blockade to distinguish lesions of the sensory branch of the radial nerve from lesions involving the lateral antebrachial cutaneous nerve.

DIFFERENTIAL DIAGNOSIS

Cheiralgia paresthetica is often misdiagnosed as lateral antebrachial cutaneous nerve syndrome. Cheiralgia paresthetica should also be differentiated from cervical radiculopathy involving the C6 or C7 roots, although patients with cervical radiculopathy will generally present not only with pain and numbness but also with reflex and motor changes. Furthermore, it should be remembered that cervical radiculopathy and radial nerve entrapment may coexist as the "double crush" syndrome. The double crush syndrome is seen most commonly with median

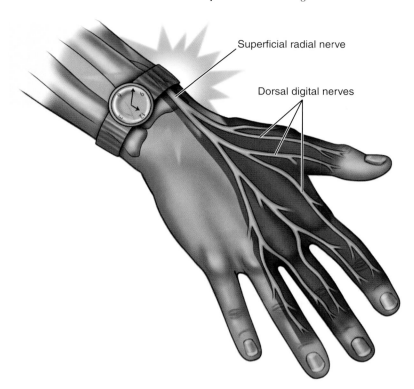

Figure 25–1. Cheiralgia paresthetica presents as pain, paresthesias, and numbness of the radial aspect of the dorsum of the hand to the base of the thumb.

nerve entrapment at the wrist or carpal tunnel syndrome.

TREATMENT

The first step in the treatment of cheiralgia paresthetica is the removal of the cause of pressure on the radial nerve. A trial of the nonsteroidal anti-inflammatory agents or the cyclooxygenase-2 (COX-2) inhibitors represents a reasonable next step. For patients for whom these treatment modalities fail, injection of the sensory branch of the radial nerve at the wrist with a local anesthetic and steroid should be considered. For persistent symptoms, surgical exploration and decompression of the nerve are indicated.

SIDE EFFECTS AND COMPLICATIONS

Radial nerve block at the wrist is a relatively safe block, with the major complications being inadvertent intravascular injection and persistent paresthesia secondary to needle trauma to the nerve. This technique can safely be performed in the presence of anticoagulation by using a 25- or 27-gauge needle, albeit at increased risk of hematoma, if the clinical situation dictates a favorable risk-to-benefit ratio. These complications can be decreased if manual pressure is applied to the area of the block immediately after injection. Application of cold packs for 20-minute periods after the block will also decrease the amount of postprocedure pain and bleeding the patient may experience.

CLINICAL PEARLS

Radial nerve block at the wrist is an effective treatment for the symptoms of cheiralgia paresthetica. Careful neurological examination to identify preexisting neurological deficits that may later be attributed to the nerve block should be performed in all patients before beginning radial nerve block at the wrist when treating cheiralgia paresthetica. If cheiralgia paresthetica is identified early, removal of the offending pressure as well as radial nerve block with a local anesthetic and steroid should lead to marked improvement in the vast majority of patients.

26 *Secretan's Syndrome*

ICD-9 CODE 782.3

THE CLINICAL SYNDROME

Secretan's syndrome, also known as *post-traumatic edema syndrome,* is caused by a peritendinous fibrosis that occurs after trauma to the dorsum of the hand. Often, the trauma is seemingly minor such as hitting the back of the hand on the corner of a desk. Initially, the swelling and tenderness may be attributed to the trauma, but instead of improvement with time, the dorsum of the hand becomes more indurated with the edema becoming brawny. Without treatment, peritendinous fibrosis and an almost myxedematous hardening of the soft tissues of the dorsum of the hand occur (Fig. 26–1). Like the pain of Dupuytren's contracture, the pain of Secretan's syndrome seems to burn itself out as the disease progresses.

SIGNS AND SYMPTOMS

Brawny edema with associated loss of extensor function of the hand following seemingly minor trauma is the sine qua non of Secretan's syndrome. Unlike reflex sympathetic dystrophy, which can mimic Secretan's syndrome, there are no sudomotor, vasomotor, or trophic nail changes, although the skin changes can appear identical to those of reflex sympathetic dystrophy.

TESTING

Plain radiographs are indicated in all patients who present with Secretan's syndrome to rule out underlying occult bony pathology. Based on the patient's clinical presentation, additional testing including complete blood cell count, uric acid, sedimentation rate, and antinuclear antibody testing may be indicated. Magnetic resonance imaging (MRI) of the hand is indicated if joint instability, infection, or tumor is suspected. Electromyography is indicated if coexistent ulnar or carpal tunnel is suspected. Injection of the areas of fibrosis will provide improvement of the pain and disability of this disease if implemented early.

DIFFERENTIAL DIAGNOSIS

Coexistent arthritis, gout of the metacarpal and interphalangeal joints, and tendinitis may also coexist with Secretan's syndrome and exacerbate the pain and disability of Secretan's syndrome. Reflex sympathetic dystrophy may present in a similar clinical manner but can be distinguished from Secretan's syndrome by the fact that the pain of reflex sympathetic dystrophy will respond to sympathetic neural blockade and the pain of Secretan's syndrome will not.

TREATMENT

Initial treatment of the pain and functional disability associated with Secretan's syndrome should include a combination of the nonsteroidal anti-inflammatory agents or cyclooxygenase-2 (COX-2) inhibitors and physical therapy. The local application of heat and cold may also be beneficial. For patients who do not respond to these treatment modalities, an injection of a local anesthetic and steroid into the areas of the peritendinous fibrosis may be a reasonable next step. The use of physical therapy, including gentle range of motion exercises, should be introduced several days after the patient undergoes this injection technique. Vigorous exercises should be avoided because they will exacerbate the patient's symptomatology.

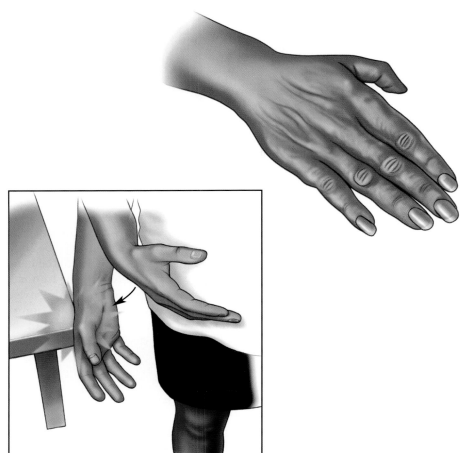

Figure 26–1. Secretan's syndrome is caused by a peritendinous fibrosis that occurs after trauma to the dorsum of the hand.

SIDE EFFECTS AND COMPLICATIONS

Injection of the peritendinous fibrosis responsible for Secretan's syndrome is a relatively safe technique if the clinician is attentive to detail. Such tendons may rupture if directly injected, and needle position should be confirmed outside the tendon before injection to avoid this complication. Another complication of this injection technique is infection. This complication should be exceedingly rare if strict aseptic technique is adhered to. Approximately 25% of patients will complain of a transient increase in pain after this injection technique and should be warned of such.

CLINICAL PEARLS

This injection technique is extremely effective in the treatment of pain and dysfunction secondary to Secretan's syndrome. Coexistent arthritis, tendinitis, and gout may also contribute to the pain and may require additional treatment with more localized injection of a local anesthetic and depot steroid. This technique is a safe procedure if careful attention is paid to the clinically relevant anatomy in the areas to be injected. Care must be taken to use sterile technique to avoid infection, as well as the use of universal precautions to avoid risk to the operator. The incidence of ecchymosis and hematoma formation can be decreased if pressure is placed on the injection site immediately after injection. The use of physical modalities, including local heat, massage, as well as gentle range of motion exercises, should be introduced several days after the patient undergoes this injection technique. Vigorous exercises should be avoided because they will exacerbate the patient's symptomatology. Simple analgesics and nonsteroidal anti-inflammatory agents may be used concurrently with this injection technique.

27 *Foreign Body Synovitis*

ICD-9 CODE 727.00

THE CLINICAL SYNDROME

Foreign body synovitis is an uncommon cause of joint or soft tissue pain encountered in clinical practice. Although foreign body synovitis can occur anywhere in the body when a foreign material is introduced into or near a joint, tendon sheath, or soft tissue surrounding a joint, the hand is most often affected. When this occurs, a chronic, inflammatory monarthritis or tenosynovitis results. Plant thorns, wood splinters, glass, and sea urchin spines are most commonly implicated.

After the initial injury, the patient suffering from foreign body tenosynovitis may note localized pain in and around the joint. If the patient realizes a foreign body is present, he or she may try to remove it. If a portion of the foreign body is left behind, foreign body synovitis can occur. After the acute injury, there may be a period of quiescence lasting weeks to months. Following this latent period, the patient will begin to experience pain and loss of function in the area of the retained foreign body, and an inflammatory monarthritis or tenosynovitis may result.

SIGNS AND SYMPTOMS

The diagnosis of foreign body synovitis is easy if the antecedent trauma is recognized. However, this is not usually the case. The patient with foreign body synovitis will present with a localized monarthritis or synovitis without obvious cause (Fig. 27–1). The patient may also complain of myalgias or flu-like symptoms in some cases. Examination of other joints will fail to reveal evidence of inflammatory arthritis and the targeted history will be negative. It will be a high index of suspicion combined with appropriate testing that will lead the clinician to a correct diagnosis.

TESTING

Magnetic resonance imaging (MRI) of the affected joint often reveals the offending foreign body. Vegetable matter such as plant thorns as well as glass are not radiopaque and will not show up on plain radiographs; failure to obtain MRI will result in a missed diagnosis. Sea urchin spines have a high calcium content and may appear on plain radiographs. Based on the patient's clinical presentation, additional testing including complete blood cell count, uric acid, sedimentation rate, and antinuclear antibody testing may be indicated. Electromyography is indicated if coexistent ulnar or carpal tunnel is suspected. Joint aspiration and synovial biopsy may be required to make the diagnosis of foreign body synovitis. Arthroscopy or arthrotomy may be the mechanism by which the diagnosis is finally made.

DIFFERENTIAL DIAGNOSIS

Again, it is the recognition of the possibility of antecedent trauma with the introduction of a foreign body that will make the diagnosis apparent. Foreign body synovitis must be distinguished from other causes of monarthritis and synovitis. Table 27–1 lists some of the common causes of monarthritis. The ultimate differential diagnosis will usually require a careful targeted history and physical examination combined with appropriate laboratory and radiographic testing.

TREATMENT

Initial treatment of the pain and functional disability associated with foreign body synovitis should include a combination of the nonsteroidal anti-

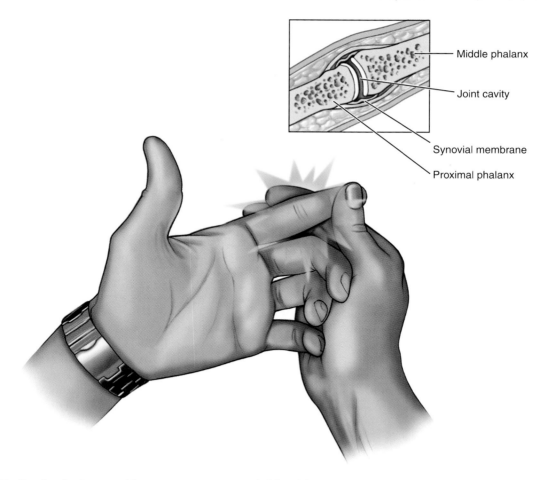

Figure 27–1. Foreign body synovitis presents as a monarthritis without apparent cause.

Table 27-1. Some Common Causes of Monarthritis

• Gout	• Amyloidosis
• Traumatic arthritis	• Osteoarthritis
• Gonococcal arthritis	• Osteonecrosis
• Charcot's joint	• Villonodular synovitis
• Other crystal arthritis	• Neoplasm
• Sarcoidosis	• Foreign body synovitis

inflammatory agents or cyclooxygenase-2 (COX-2) inhibitors and physical therapy. The local application of heat and cold may also be beneficial. For patients who do not respond to these treatment modalities, an injection into the affected area with a local anesthetic and steroid may be a reasonable next step. The use of physical therapy, including gentle range of motion exercises, should be introduced several days after the patient undergoes this injection technique. Vigorous exercises should be avoided because they will exacerbate the patient's symptomatology. Surgical removal of the offending foreign body will often be the only intervention that will successfully treat foreign body synovitis.

SIDE EFFECTS AND COMPLICATIONS

The main complication associated with foreign body synovitis is the risk of permanent joint damage due to delayed diagnosis. Injection of the area of synovitis syndrome is a relatively safe technique if the clinician is attentive to detail. Inflamed tendons may rupture if directly injected, and needle position should be confirmed outside the tendon before injection to avoid this complication. Another complication of this injection technique is infection. This complication should be exceedingly rare if strict aseptic technique is adhered to. Approximately 25% of patients will complain of a transient increase in pain after this injection technique and should be warned of such.

CLINICAL PEARLS

The diagnosis of foreign body synovitis is easy if the clinician thinks of it. By including foreign body synovitis in the differential diagnosis of patients suffering from monarthritis or tenosynovitis, the diagnosis will be more easily recognized. The early use of MRI of the affected area also helps increase the diagnostic accuracy of the clinician.

28 Glomus Tumor of the Hand

ICD-9 CODE 228.00

THE CLINICAL SYNDROME

Glomus tumor of the hand is an uncommon cause of distal finger pain. It is the result of tumor formation of the glomus body, which is a neuromyoarterial apparatus whose function is to regulate peripheral blood flow in the digits. The majority of patients suffering from glomus tumor are women between the ages of 30 and 50 years. The pain is very severe in intensity and is lancinating and boring in nature. The tumor frequently involves the nail bed and may invade the distal phalanx. Patients suffering from glomus tumor of the hand will exhibit the classic triad of excruciating distal finger pain, cold intolerance, and tenderness to palpation of the affected digit.

Multiple glomus tumors are present in approximately 25% of patients diagnosed with this disease. Glomus tumors can also occur in the foot and, occasionally, in other parts of the body.

SIGNS AND SYMPTOMS

The diagnosis of glomus tumor of the hand is based primarily on three points in the patient's clinical history: (1) excruciating pain that is localized to a distal digit; (2) the ability to trigger the pain by palpating the area; and (3) marked intolerance to cold. The pain of glomus tumor can be reproduced by placing the affected digit in a glass of ice water. If glomus tumor is present, the characteristic lancinating, boring pain will occur within 30 to 60 seconds. Placing other unaffected fingers of the same hand in ice water will not trigger the pain in the affected finger. Nail bed ridging is present in many patients with glomus tumor of the hand, and a small blue or dark red spot at the base of the nail is visible in 10% to 15% of patients suffering from the disease (Fig. 28–1). The patient with glomus tumor of the hand will frequently wear a finger protector on the affected digit and will guard against hitting the digit on anything to avoid triggering the pain.

TESTING

Magnetic resonance imaging (MRI) of the affected digit often reveals the actual glomus tumor and may also reveal erosion or a perforating lesion of the phalanx beneath the tumor. The tumor will appear as a very high and homogeneous signal on T2-weighted images. The bony changes associated with glomus tumor of the hand may also appear on plain radiographs if a careful comparison of the corresponding contralateral digit is made. Radionuclide bone scan may also reveal localized bony destruction. The ice water test mentioned earlier will help the clinician strengthen his or her diagnosis. Based on the patient's clinical presentation, additional testing including complete blood cell count, uric acid, sedimentation rate, and antinuclear antibody testing may be indicated. Electromyography is indicated if coexistent ulnar or carpal tunnel is suspected. Surgical exploration of the affected digit and nail bed will often be necessary to confirm the diagnosis.

DIFFERENTIAL DIAGNOSIS

The triad of localized excruciating distal digit pain, tenderness to palpation, and cold intolerance will make the diagnosis apparent to the astute clinician. Glomus tumor of the hand must be distinguished from other causes of localized hand pain, including subungual melanoma and osteoid osteoma. If a history of trauma is present, fracture, osteomyelitis, tenosynovitis, and foreign body synovitis should be considered. If there is no history of trauma, then gout,

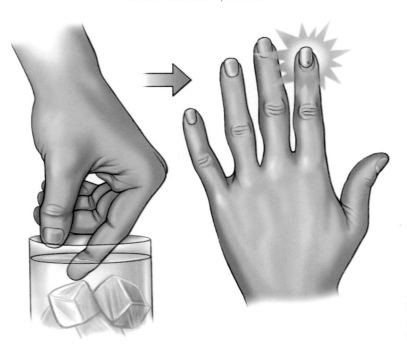

Figure 28–1. Glomus tumor is characterized by (1) excruciating distal digit pain, (2) ability to trigger the pain by palpation, and (3) marked intolerance to cold.

the other crystal monoarthropathies, tumors, and diseases of the nail and nail bed should be considered. Reflex sympathetic dystrophy should be distinguishable from glomus tumor of the hand because the pain of reflex sympathetic dystrophy is less localized and is associated with trophic skin and nail changes and vasomotor and sudomotor abnormalities. Raynaud's syndrome usually involves the entire hand, and the ice water test mentioned will usually trigger pain if the "unaffected" finger is tested.

TREATMENT

The mainstay of treatment of glomus tumor is surgical removal. Medication management is uniformly disappointing. Injection of the affected digit in the point of maximal tenderness may provide temporary relief of the pain of glomus tumor and will block the positive ice water test response, further strengthening the diagnosis.

SIDE EFFECTS AND COMPLICATIONS

The main complication associated with glomus tumor of the hand involves the problems associated with delayed diagnosis, mainly ongoing destruction of the bone and nail bed. Although usually localized and well encapsulated, rarely, these tumors can exhibit aggressive invasive tendencies, making complete excision of the tumor and careful follow-up mandatory.

CLINICAL PEARLS

The diagnosis of glomus tumor of the hand is usually straightforward if the clinician identifies the unique nature of its clinical presentation. Because of the rare potential for aggressive, invasive behavior, complete excision and careful follow-up are important.

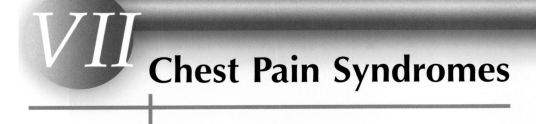

VII Chest Pain Syndromes

29 *Devil's Grip*

ICD-9 CODE 074.1

THE CLINICAL SYNDROME

Devil's grip is an uncommon cause of chest pain. Also known as *Bornholm's disease, dry pleurisy,* and *Sylvest's disease,* devil's grip is caused by acute infection with coxsackievirus. This virus is transmitted via the fecal-oral route and is highly contagious, owing to a long period of viral shedding of up to 6 weeks. In some patients, their immune system limits the infection to a mild fever or flu-like illness called *summer fever.* However, in others, a full-fledged infection with resultant pleurodynia and cough develops.

There is a seasonal variation to occurrence of devil's grip, with 90% of cases occurring in the summer and fall with August being the peak month. There is no gender predilection, but the disease occurs more commonly in young adults and, occasionally, in children. The pain is severe in intensity and is described as sharp or pleuritic in character. The pain occurs in paroxysms that can last up to 30 minutes.

SIGNS AND SYMPTOMS

Physical examination of the patient suffering from devil's grip will reveal a patient who appears acutely ill (Fig. 29–1). Pallor and fever are invariably present, as is tachycardia. Patients may complain of malaise, sore throat, and arthralgia, which may confuse the clinical picture. Examination of the chest wall reveals minimal physical findings, although a friction rub is sometimes present. During the paroxysms of pain, the patient suffering from devil's grip will attempt to splint or protect the affected area. Deep inspiration or movement of the chest wall will markedly increase the pain of devil's grip.

DIFFERENTIAL DIAGNOSIS

As is the case with costochondritis, costosternal joint pain, Tietze's syndrome, and rib fractures, a significant number of patients who suffer from devil's grip first seek medical attention because they believe they are suffering a heart attack. If the area innervated by the subcostal nerve is involved, patients may believe they are suffering from gallbladder disease. Statistically, children suffering from devil's grip suffer from abdominal pain more often than do adults, and such pain may be attributed to appendicitis, leading to unnecessary surgery. In contradistinction to most other causes of pain involving the chest wall, which are musculoskeletal or neuropathic in nature, the pain of devil's grip is infectious in nature. The constitutional symptoms associated with devil's grip may lead the clinician to consider pneumonia, empyema, and, on occasion, pulmonary embolus as the most likely diagnosis.

TESTING

Plain radiographs are indicated in all patients who present with pain thought to be the result of infection with coxsackievirus to rule out occult chest wall pathology, pulmonary tumors, pneumonia, or empyema. Ventilation-perfusion studies of the lungs are indicated if pulmonary embolism is being considered in the differential diagnosis. Based on the patient's clinical presentation, additional testing including complete blood cell count, sedimentation rate, and throat cultures for *Streptococcus* may be indicated. Computed tomography (CT) scan of the thoracic contents is indicated if occult mass or empyema is suspected.

DIFFERENTIAL DIAGNOSIS

As mentioned, the pain of devil's grip is often mistaken for pain of cardiac or gallbladder origin and

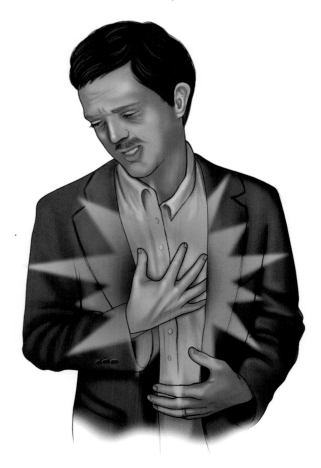

Figure 29–1. Deep inspiration markedly increases the pain of devil's grip.

can lead to visits to the emergency department and unnecessary cardiac and gastrointestinal work-ups. If trauma has occurred, devil's grip may coexist with fractured ribs or fractures of the sternum itself, which can be missed on plain radiographs and may require radionucleotide bone scanning for proper identification. Tietze's syndrome, which is painful enlargement of the upper costochondral cartilage associated with viral infection, can be confused with devil's grip.

Neuropathic pain involving the chest wall may also be confused or coexist with costosternal syndrome. Examples of such neuropathic pain include diabetic polyneuropathies and acute herpes zoster involving the thoracic nerves. The possibility of diseases of the structures of the mediastinum remains ever present and at times can be difficult to diagnose. Pathological processes that inflame the pleura, such as pulmonary embolus, infection, and tumor, also need to be considered.

TREATMENT

Initial treatment of devil's grip should include a combination of simple analgesics and the nonsteroidal anti-inflammatory agents or cyclooxygenase-2 (COX-2) inhibitors. If these medications do not adequately control the patient's symptomatology, opioid analgesics may be added during the period of acute pain.

The local application of heat and cold may also be beneficial to provide symptomatic relief of the pain of devil's grip. The use of an elastic rib belt may also help provide symptomatic relief in some patients. For patients who do not respond to these treatment modalities, the following injection technique using a local anesthetic and steroid may be a reasonable next step.

The patient is placed in the prone position with the patient's arms hanging loosely off the side of the cart. Alternatively, this block can be done in the sitting or lateral position. The rib to be blocked is identified by palpating its path at the posterior axillary line. The index and middle fingers are then placed on the rib bracketing the site of needle insertion. The skin is then prepped with antiseptic solution. A 22-gauge $1\frac{1}{2}$-inch needle is attached to a 12-mL syringe and is advanced perpendicular to the skin, aiming for the middle of the rib between the index and middle finger. The needle should impinge on bone after being advanced approximately $\frac{3}{4}$ inch. After bony contact is made, the needle is withdrawn into the subcutaneous tissues and the skin and subcutaneous tissues are retracted with the palpating fingers inferiorly. This allows the needle to be walked off the inferior margin of the rib. As soon as bony contact is lost, the needle is slowly advanced approximately 2 mm deeper. This will place the needle in proximity to the costal groove, which contains the intercostal nerve as well as the intercostal artery and vein (Fig. 29–2). After careful aspiration reveals no blood or air, 3 to 5 mL of 1.0% preservative-free lidocaine is injected. If there is an inflammatory component to the pain, the local anesthetic is combined with 80 mg of methylprednisolone and is injected in incremental doses. Subsequent daily nerve blocks are carried out in a similar manner, substituting 40 mg of methylprednisolone for the initial 80-mg dose. Because of the overlapping innervation of the chest and upper abdominal wall, the intercostal nerves above and below the nerve suspected of subserving the painful condition will have to be blocked.

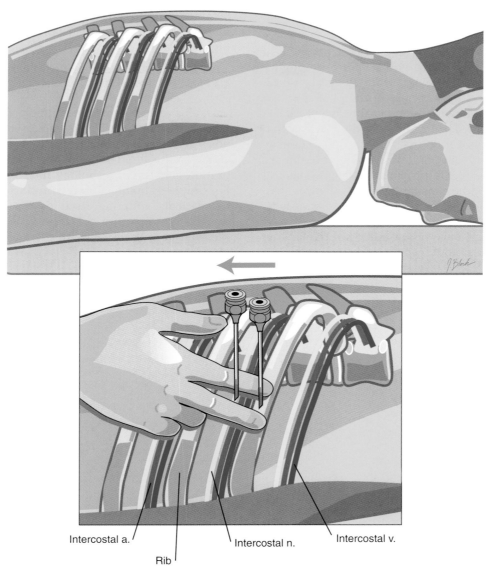

Intercostal a.

Rib

Intercostal n.

Intercostal v.

Figure 29–2

COMPLICATIONS AND PITFALLS

The major problem in the care of patients thought to suffer from devil's grip is the failure to identify potentially serious pathology of the thorax or upper abdomen. Given the proximity of the pleural space, pneumothorax following intercostal nerve block is a distinct possibility. The incidence of the complication is less than 1%, but it occurs with greater frequency in patients with chronic obstructive pulmonary disease. Because of the proximity to the intercostal nerve and artery, the clinician should carefully calculate the total milligram dosage of local anesthetic administered as vascular uptake via these vessels is high. Although uncommon, infection remains an ever-present possibility, especially in the immuno-compromised patient with cancer. Early detection of infection is crucial to avoid potentially life-threatening sequelae.

CLINICAL PEARLS

Devil's grip is an uncommon cause of chest pain that is frequently misdiagnosed. Correct diagnosis is necessary to properly treat this painful condition and to avoid overlooking serious intrathoracic or intra-abdominal pathology. Intercostal nerve block is a simple technique that can produce dramatic relief for patients suffering from devil's grip. As mentioned, the proximity of the intercostal nerve to the pleural space makes careful attention to technique mandatory.

30 *Sternoclavicular Syndrome*

ICD-9 CODE 786.59

THE CLINICAL SYNDROME

With the advent of seat belts that cross the chest, sternoclavicular syndrome is being seen with greater frequency by clinicians. The joint is often traumatized during acceleration/deceleration injuries and blunt trauma to the chest. With severe trauma the joint may sublux or dislocate. Overuse or misuse can also result in acute inflammation of the sternoclavicular joint, which can be quite debilitating for the patient. Because the sternoclavicular joint is a true joint, it is susceptible to the development of arthritis, including osteoarthritis, rheumatoid arthritis, ankylosing spondylitis, Reiter's syndrome, and psoriatic arthritis. The joint is also subject to invasion by tumor either from primary malignancies, including thymoma, or from metastatic disease. Pain emanating from the sternoclavicular joint often mimics the pain of cardiac origin.

SIGNS AND SYMPTOMS

Physical examination will reveal that the patient vigorously attempts to splint the joint by keeping the shoulders stiffly in neutral position (Fig. 30–1). Pain is reproduced with active protraction or retraction of the shoulder as well as full elevation of the arm. Shrugging of the shoulder may also reproduce the pain. The sternoclavicular joint may be tender to palpation and feel hot and swollen if acutely inflamed. The patient may also complain of a clicking sensation with movement of the joint.

TESTING

Plain radiographs are indicated in all patients who present with pain thought to be emanating from the sternoclavicular joint to rule out occult bony pathology, including tumor. Based on the patient's clinical presentation, additional testing including complete blood cell count, prostate specific antigen, sedimentation rate, and antinuclear antibody testing may be indicated. Magnetic resonance imaging (MRI) of the joint is indicated if joint instability is suspected. Injection of the sternoclavicular joint with a local anesthetic and/or steroid serves as both a diagnostic and therapeutic maneuver.

DIFFERENTIAL DIAGNOSIS

As mentioned, the pain of sternoclavicular syndrome is often mistaken for pain of cardiac origin and can lead to visits to the emergency department and unnecessary cardiac work-ups. If trauma has occurred, sternoclavicular syndrome may coexist with fractured ribs or fractures of the sternum itself, which can be missed on plain radiographs and may require radionucleotide bone scanning for proper identification. Tietze's syndrome, which is painful enlargement of the upper costochondral cartilage associated with viral infections, can be confused with sternoclavicular syndrome.

Neuropathic pain involving the chest wall may also be confused or coexist with sternoclavicular syndrome. Examples of such neuropathic pain include diabetic polyneuropathies and acute herpes zoster involving the thoracic nerves. The possibility of diseases of the structures of the mediastinum remains ever present and at times can be difficult to diagnose. Pathological processes that inflame the pleura, such as pulmonary embolus, infection, and Bornholm's disease, also need to be considered.

TREATMENT

Initial treatment of the pain and functional disability associated with sternoclavicular syndrome should

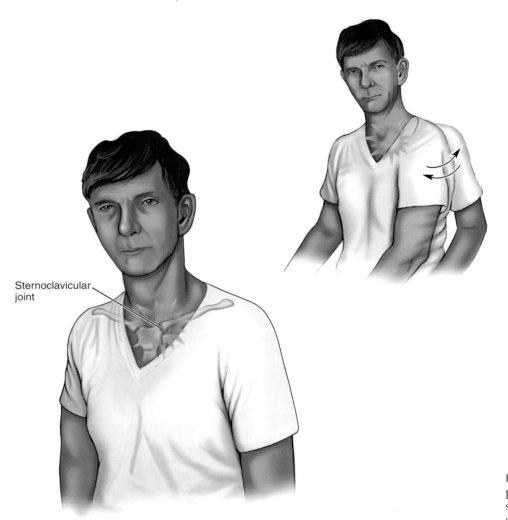

Sternoclavicular
joint

Figure 30–1. Acute
protraction or retraction of the
shoulder reproduces the pain
of sternoclavicular syndrome.

include a combination of the nonsteroidal anti-inflammatory agents or the cyclooxygenase-2 (COX-2) inhibitors. The local application of heat and cold may also be beneficial. The use of an elastic clavicle splint may also help provide symptomatic relief and help protect the sternoclavicular joints from additional trauma. For patients who do not respond to these treatment modalities, injection of the sternoclavicular joint using a local anesthetic and steroid may be a reasonable next step.

COMPLICATIONS AND PITFALLS

Because of the many pathological processes that may mimic the pain of sternoclavicular syndrome, the clinician must be careful to rule out underlying cardiac disease and diseases of the lung and structures of the mediastinum. Failure to do so could lead to disastrous results. The major complication of the above injection technique is pneumothorax if the needle is placed too laterally or deeply and invades the pleural space. Infection, although rare, can occur if strict aseptic technique is not adhered to. The possibility of trauma to the contents of the mediastinum remains an ever-present possibility. This complica-

tion can be greatly decreased if the clinician plays close attention to accurate needle placement.

CLINICAL PEARLS

Patients suffering from pain emanating from the sternoclavicular joint will often attribute their pain symptomatology to a heart attack. Reassurance is required although it should be remembered that this musculoskeletal pain syndrome and coronary artery disease can coexist. Tietze's syndrome, which is painful enlargement of the upper costochondral cartilage associated with viral infections, can be confused with sternoclavicular syndrome, although both respond to the injection technique described. The use of physical modalities, including local heat as well as gentle range of motion exercises, should be introduced several days after the patient undergoes this injection technique for sternoclavicular joint pain. Vigorous exercises should be avoided because they will exacerbate the patient's symptomatology. Simple analgesics and nonsteroidal anti-inflammatory agents may be used concurrently with this injection technique. Laboratory evaluation for collagen vascular disease is indicated in patients suffering from sternoclavicular joint pain in whom other joints are involved.

31 Postmastectomy Pain

ICD-9 CODE 611.71

THE CLINICAL SYNDROME

Postmastectomy pain syndrome is a constellation of symptoms that include pain in the anterior chest, breast, axilla, and medial upper extremity after surgical procedures on the breast. *Postmastectomy pain* is somewhat of a misnomer in that the clinical syndrome includes the pain mentioned here even if the patient has only a lumpectomy or if another less-extensive surgical procedure is performed on the breast. The pain is often described as constricting with a continuing dull ache. In addition to these symptoms, many patients with postmastectomy pain syndrome will also complain of sudden paresthesia radiating into the breast and/or axilla. In some patients, a burning, allodynic pain reminiscent of reflex sympathetic dystrophy may be the principal complaint. The intensity of postmastectomy pain is moderate to severe. It is important to note that the onset of postmastectomy pain may occur immediately after surgery and initially be confused with the expected postsurgical pain, or the onset may be more insidious, occurring gradually 2 to 6 weeks after the inciting surgical procedure. If complete mastectomy is performed, phantom breast pain may further confound the diagnosis, as may associated lymphedema. Sleep disturbance is a common finding in patients suffering from postmastectomy pain.

SIGNS AND SYMPTOMS

Evaluation of the patient suffering from postmastectomy syndrome requires that the clinician take a careful history designed to delineate the various components that make up the patient's pain to help guide the physical examination. The clinician should question the patient specifically about the presence of phantom breast pain, which may be quite distressing to the patient when superimposed on the pain of postmastectomy syndrome.

Typical physical findings in patients suffering from postmastectomy syndrome include areas of decreased sensation, hyperpathia, and dysesthesia in the distribution of the intercostalbrachial nerve, which is a branch of the second intercostal nerve (Fig. 31–1). This nerve is frequently damaged during breast surgery. Allodynia outside the distribution of the intercostalbrachial nerve is also often present. Movement of the arm and axilla will often exacerbate the pain, which leads to splinting and disuse of the affected shoulder and upper extremity. This disuse will often worsen any lymphedema that is present. If the disuse of the upper extremity continues, frozen shoulder may develop, further complicating the clinical picture.

The clinician should always be alert to the possibility of metastatic disease or direct extension of tumor into the chest wall, which may mimic the pain of postmastectomy syndrome.

The findings of the targeted history and physical examination will assist the clinician to make an assessment of the sympathetic, neuropathic, and musculoskeletal components of the pain and design a rational treatment plan.

TESTING

Plain radiographs are indicated in all patients who present with pain thought to be due to postmastectomy syndrome to rule out occult bony pathology, including tumor. Electromyography will help rule out damage to the intercostalbrachial nerve or plexopathy that may be contributing to the patient's pain. Radionucleotide bone scanning may be useful to rule out occult pathological fractures of the ribs and/or sternum. Based on the patient's clinical presentation, additional testing including complete blood cell

require radionucleotide bone scanning for proper identification.

Neuropathic pain involving the chest wall may also be confused or coexist with postmastectomy syndrome. Examples of such neuropathic pain include diabetic polyneuropathies and acute herpes zoster involving the thoracic nerves. The possibility of diseases of the structures of the mediastinum remains ever present and at times can be difficult to diagnose. Pathological processes that inflame the pleura, such as pulmonary embolus, infection, and Bornholm's disease, may also mimic the pain of postmastectomy syndrome.

TREATMENT

Initial treatment of postmastectomy syndrome should include a combination of simple analgesics and the nonsteroidal anti-inflammatory agents or the cyclooxygenase-2 (COX-2) inhibitors. If these medications do not adequately control the patient's symptomatology, a tricyclic antidepressant or gabapentin should be added.

Traditionally, the tricyclic antidepressants have been a mainstay in the palliation of pain secondary to postmastectomy syndrome. Controlled studies have demonstrated the efficacy of amitriptyline for this indication. Other tricyclic antidepressants including nortriptyline and desipramine have also shown to be clinically useful. Unfortunately, this class of drugs is associated with significant anticholinergic side effects, including dry mouth, constipation, sedation, and urinary retention. These drugs should be used with caution in those suffering from glaucoma, cardiac arrhythmia, and prostatism. To minimize side effects and encourage compliance, the primary care physician should start amitriptyline or nortriptyline at a 10-mg dose at bedtime. The dose can be then titrated upward to 25 mg at bedtime as side effects allow. Upward titration of dosage in 25-mg increments can be carried out each week as side effects allow. Even at lower doses, patients will generally report a rapid improvement in sleep disturbance and will begin to experience some pain relief in 10 to 14 days. If the patient does not experience any improvement in pain as the dose is being titrated upward, the addition of gabapentin alone or in combination with nerve blocks of the intercostal nerves with local anesthetics and/or steroid is recommended. The selective serotonin reuptake inhibitors such as fluoxetine have also been used to treat the pain of diabetic neuropathy, and although better tolerated than the tricyclic antidepressants, they appear to be less efficacious.

If the antidepressant compounds are ineffective or contraindicated, gabapentin represents a reasonable

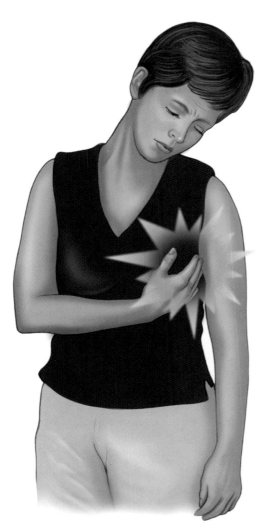

Figure 31–1. The pain of postmastectomy syndrome is due to damage of the intercostalbrachial nerve.

count, prostate specific antigen, sedimentation rate, and antinuclear antibody testing may be indicated. Computed tomography (CT) scan of the thoracic contents is indicated if occult mass is suspected. Magnetic resonance imaging (MRI) of the brachial plexus should also be considered if plexopathy secondary to tumor involvement is a consideration.

DIFFERENTIAL DIAGNOSIS

As mentioned, the pain of postmastectomy syndrome is often mistaken for postoperative pain. If the breast surgery was performed for malignancy, a careful search for metastatic disease or tumor invasion of the chest wall is mandatory. Postmastectomy syndrome may coexist with pathological fractured ribs or pathological fractures of the sternum itself, which can be missed on plain radiographs and may

alternative. Gabapentin should be started with a 300-mg dose of gabapentin at bedtime for 2 nights. The patient should be cautioned about potential side effects, including dizziness, sedation, confusion, and rash. The drug is then increased in 300-mg increments, given in equally divided doses over 2 days, as side effects allow until pain relief is obtained or a total dose of 2400 mg daily is reached. At this point, if the patient has experienced partial relief of pain, blood values are measured and the drug is carefully titrated upward using 100-mg tablets. Rarely will more than 3600 mg daily be required.

The local application of heat and cold may also be beneficial to provide symptomatic relief of the pain of postmastectomy syndrome. The use of an elastic rib belt may also help provide symptomatic relief. For patients who do not respond to these treatment modalities, injection of the affected intercostal nerves or thoracic epidural nerve block using local anesthetic and steroid may be a reasonable next step.

COMPLICATIONS AND PITFALLS

The major problem in the care of patients thought to suffer from postmastectomy syndrome is the failure to identify potentially serious pathology of the thorax or upper abdomen due to metastatic disease or invasion of the chest wall and thorax by tumor. Given the proximity of the pleural space, pneumothorax following intercostal nerve block is a distinct possibility. The incidence of the complication is less than 1%, but it occurs with greater frequency in patients with chronic obstructive pulmonary disease. Although uncommon, infection remains an ever-present possibility, especially in the immunocompromised patient with cancer. Early detection of infection is crucial to avoid potentially life-threatening sequelae.

CLINICAL PEARLS

Postmastectomy syndrome is a cause of chest wall and thoracic pain that should not be overlooked in patients after breast surgery. Correct diagnosis is necessary to properly treat this painful condition and to avoid overlooking serious intrathoracic or intraabdominal pathology. The use of the pharmacological agents mentioned, including gabapentin, will allow the clinician to adequately control the pain of postmastectomy syndrome. Intercostal nerve block is a simple technique that can produce dramatic relief for patients suffering from postmastectomy syndrome. As mentioned, the proximity of the intercostal nerve to the pleural space makes careful attention to technique mandatory.

32 *Sternalis Syndrome*

ICD-9 CODE 786.52

THE CLINICAL SYNDROME

Chest wall pain syndromes are commonly encountered in clinical practice. Some occur with relatively greater frequency and are more readily identified by the clinician, such as costochondritis and Tietze's syndrome. Others occur so infrequently that they are often misdiagnosed, resulting in less-than-optimal outcome. Sternalis syndrome is one such infrequent cause of anterior chest wall pain. Sternalis is a constellation symptoms consisting of midline anterior chest wall that can radiate to the retrosternal area and the medial aspect of the arm. Sternalis syndrome can mimic the pain of myocardial infarction and is frequently misdiagnosed as such. Sternalis syndrome is a myofascial pain syndrome and is characterized by trigger points in the midsternal area. In contradistinction to costosternal syndrome, which also presents as midsternal pain, the pain of sternalis syndrome is not exacerbated by movement of the chest wall and shoulder. The intensity of the pain associated with sternalis syndrome is mild to moderate and described as having a deep, aching character. The pain of sternalis syndrome is intermittent.

SIGNS AND SYMPTOMS

On physical examination, the patient suffering from sternalis syndrome will exhibit myofascial trigger points at the midline over the sternum (Fig. 32–1). Occasionally, there is a coexistent trigger point in the pectoralis muscle or sternal head of the sternocleidomastoid muscle. Pain is reproduced with palpation of these trigger points rather than movement of the chest wall and shoulders. A positive jump sign will be present when these trigger points are stimulated. Trigger points at the lateral border of the scapula may also be present and amenable to injection therapy. As mentioned, movement of the shoulders and chest wall will not exacerbate the pain.

TESTING

Plain radiographs are indicated in all patients who present with suspected sternalis syndrome to rule out occult bony pathology, including metastatic lesions. Based on the patient's clinical presentation, additional testing including complete blood cell count, prostate specific antigen, sedimentation rate, and antinuclear antibody testing may be indicated. Magnetic resonance imaging (MRI) of the chest is indicated if a retrosternal mass such as thymoma is suspected. Electromyography is indicated in patients suffering from sternalis syndrome to help rule out cervical radiculopathy or plexopathy that may be considered due to the referred arm pain. Injection of the sternalis muscle with a local anesthetic and steroid serves as both a diagnostic and therapeutic maneuver.

DIFFERENTIAL DIAGNOSIS

As mentioned, the pain of sternalis syndrome is often mistaken for pain of cardiac origin and can lead to visits to the emergency department and unnecessary cardiac work-ups. If trauma has occurred, sternalis syndrome may coexist with fractured ribs or fractures of the sternum itself, which can be missed on plain radiographs and may require radionucleotide bone scanning for proper identification. Tietze's syndrome, which is painful enlargement of the upper costochondral cartilage associated with viral infections, can be confused with sternalis syndrome, as can costosternal syndrome.

Neuropathic pain involving the chest wall may also be confused or coexist with costosternal syndrome. Examples of such neuropathic pain include diabetic

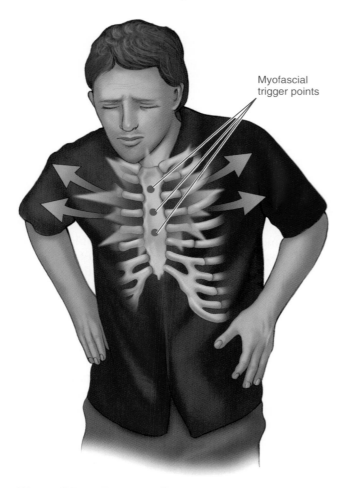

Myofascial
trigger points

Figure 32–1. Patients suffering from sternalis syndrome exhibit myofascial trigger points at the midline over the sternum.

polyneuropathies and acute herpes zoster involving the thoracic nerves. The possibility of diseases of the structures of the mediastinum remains ever present and at times can be difficult to diagnose. Pathological processes that inflame the pleura, such as pulmonary embolus, infection, and tumor, also need to be considered.

TREATMENT

Initial treatment of sternalis syndrome should include a combination of simple analgesics and the nonsteroidal anti-inflammatory agents or the cyclooxygenase-2 (COX-2) inhibitors. The local application of heat and cold may also be beneficial to provide symptomatic relief of the pain of sternalis syndrome. The use of an elastic rib belt may also help

provide symptomatic relief in some patients. For patients who do not respond to these treatment modalities, injection of the trigger areas located in the sternalis muscle using a local anesthetic and steroid may be a reasonable next step.

COMPLICATIONS AND PITFALLS

The major problem in the care of patients thought to suffer from sternalis syndrome is the failure to identify potentially serious pathology of the thorax and/or mediastinum. Given the proximity of the pleural space, pneumothorax after injection of the sternalis muscle is a distinct possibility as is injury to the mediastinal and intrathoracic structures. Approximately 25% of patients will complain of a transient increase in pain after this injection technique and should be warned of such.

CLINICAL PEARLS

Patients suffering from sternalis syndrome will often present to the emergency department, fearing they are suffering a heart attack. The syndrome is also frequently misdiagnosed as a cervical radiculopathy due to the referred arm pain. Electromyography will help delineate the etiology and extent of neural compromise.

This injection technique is extremely effective in the treatment of sternalis syndrome. Coexistent costosternal or manubriosternal arthritis may also contribute to anterior chest wall pain and may require additional treatment with a more localized injection of a local anesthetic and depot-steroid. This technique is a safe procedure if careful attention is paid to the clinically relevant anatomy in the areas to be injected. Pneumothorax can be avoided if shorter needles are used and the needle is not advanced too deeply. Care must be taken to use sterile technique to avoid infection, as well as the use of universal precautions to avoid risk to the operator. The incidence of ecchymosis and hematoma formation can be decreased if pressure is placed on the injection site immediately after injection. The use of physical modalities, including local heat as well as gentle range of motion exercises, should be introduced several days after the patient undergoes this injection technique for shoulder pain. Vigorous exercises should be avoided because they will exacerbate the patient's symptomatology. Simple analgesics and nonsteroidal anti-inflammatory agents may be used concurrently with this injection technique.

33

Slipping Rib Syndrome

ICD-9 CODE 786.59

THE CLINICAL SYNDROME

Encountered more frequently in clinical practice since the increased use of across-the-chest seat belts and air bags, slipping rib syndrome is often misdiagnosed, leading to prolonged suffering and excessive testing for intra-abdominal and intrathoracic pathology. Slipping rib syndrome is a constellation of symptoms consisting of severe knife-like pain emanating from the lower costal cartilages associated with hypermobility of the anterior end of the lower costal cartilages. The tenth rib is most commonly involved, but the eight and ninth ribs can also be affected. This syndrome is also known as *rib-tip syndrome*. Slipping rib syndrome is almost always associated with trauma to the costal cartilage of the lower ribs. These cartilages are often traumatized during acceleration/deceleration injuries and blunt trauma to the chest. With severe trauma, the cartilage may sublux or dislocate from the ribs. Patients with slipping rib syndrome may also complain of a clicking sensation with movement of the affected ribs and associated cartilage.

SIGNS AND SYMPTOMS

Physical examination will reveal that the patient will vigorously attempt to splint the affected costal cartilage joints by keeping the thoracolumbar spine slightly flexed (Fig. 33–1). Pain is reproduced with pressure on the affected costal cartilage. Patients with slipping rib syndrome exhibit a positive hooking maneuver test. The hooking maneuver test is performed by having the patient lie in the supine position with the abdominal muscles relaxed while the clinician hooks his or her fingers under the lower rib cage and pulls gently outward. Pain and a clicking or snapping sensation of the affected ribs and cartilage indicate a positive test.

TESTING

Plain radiographs are indicated in all patients who present with pain thought to be emanating from the lower costal cartilage and ribs to rule out occult bony pathology, including rib fracture and tumor. Based on the patient's clinical presentation, additional testing including complete blood cell count, prostate specific antigen, sedimentation rate, and antinuclear antibody testing may be indicated. Magnetic resonance imaging (MRI) of the affected ribs and cartilage is indicated if joint instability or occult mass is suspected. The following injection technique serves as both a diagnostic and therapeutic maneuver.

DIFFERENTIAL DIAGNOSIS

As mentioned, the pain of slipping rib syndrome is often mistaken for pain of cardiac or gallbladder origin and can lead to visits to the emergency department and unnecessary cardiac and gastrointestinal work-ups. If trauma has occurred, slipping rib syndrome may coexist with fractured ribs or fractures of the sternum itself, which can be missed on plain radiographs and may require radionucleotide bone scanning for proper identification. Tietze's syndrome, which is painful enlargement of the upper costochondral cartilage associated with viral infections, can be confused with slipping rib syndrome as can devil's grip, which is a pleura-based pain syndrome of infectious etiology.

Neuropathic pain involving the chest wall may also be confused or coexist with slipping rib syndrome. Examples of such neuropathic pain include diabetic polyneuropathies and acute herpes zoster involving the thoracic nerves. The possibility of dis-

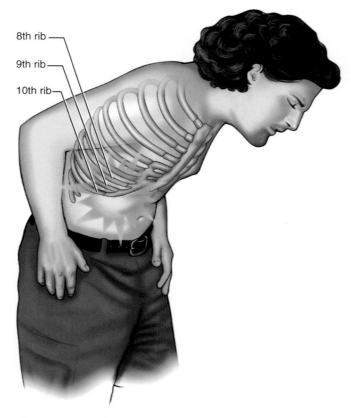

8th rib

9th rib

10th rib

Figure 33–1. Patients suffering from slipping rib syndrome exhibit pain on "hooking" of the affected costochondral cartilage.

eases of the structures of the mediastinum remains ever present and at times can be difficult to diagnose. Pathological processes that inflame the pleura, such as pulmonary embolus, infection, and tumor, also need to be considered.

TREATMENT

Initial treatment of the pain and functional disability associated with slipping rib syndrome should include a combination of the nonsteroidal anti-inflammatory agents or cyclooxygenase-2 (COX-2) inhibitors and physical therapy. The local application of heat and cold may also be beneficial. The repetitive movements that incite the syndrome should be avoided. For patients who do not respond to these treatment modalities, injection of the affected costochondral cartilages with a local anesthetic and steroid may be a reasonable next step.

To inject the slipping ribs, the patient is placed in the supine position, and proper preparation with antiseptic solution of the skin overlying the affected costal cartilage and rib is carried out. A sterile syringe

containing 1.0 mL of 0.25% preservative-free bupivacaine for each joint to be injected and 40 mg of methylprednisolone is attached to a 25-gauge 1½-inch needle using strict aseptic technique.

With strict aseptic technique, the distal rib and costal cartilage are identified. The lower margin of each affected distal rib is identified and marked with a sterile marker. The needle is then carefully advanced at the point marked through the skin and subcutaneous tissues until the needle tip impinges on the periosteum of the underlying rib. The needle is then withdrawn back into the subcutaneous tissues and walked inferiorly off the inferior rib margin. The needle should be advanced just beyond the inferior rib margin but no farther, or pneumothorax or damage to the abdominal viscera could result. After careful aspiration to ensure that the needle tip is not in an intercostal vein or artery, 1 mL of solution is gently injected. There should be limited resistance to injection. If significant resistance is encountered, the needle should be withdrawn slightly until the injection proceeds with only limited resistance. This procedure is repeated for each affected rib and associated cartilage. The needle is then removed, and a sterile pressure dressing and ice pack are placed at the injection site.

SIDE EFFECTS AND COMPLICATIONS

The major problem in the care of patients thought to suffer from slipping rib syndrome is the failure to identify potentially serious pathology of the thorax or upper abdomen. Given the proximity of the pleural space, pneumothorax following the injection technique described is a distinct possibility. The incidence of the complication is less than 1%, but it occurs with greater frequency in patients with chronic obstructive pulmonary disease. Because of the proximity to the intercostal nerve and artery, the clinician should carefully calculate the total milligram dosage of local anesthetic administered because vascular uptake via these vessels is high. Although uncommon, infection remains an ever-present possibility, especially in the immuno-compromised patient with cancer. Early detection of infection is crucial to avoid potentially life-threatening sequelae.

CLINICAL PEARLS

Patients suffering from pain emanating from slipping rib often attribute their pain symptomatology to a gallbladder attack or ulcer disease. Reassurance is required, although it should be remembered that this musculoskeletal pain syndrome and intra-abdominal pathology can coexist. Care must be taken to use sterile technique to avoid infection, as well as the use of universal precautions to avoid risk to the operator. The incidence of ecchymosis and hematoma formation can be decreased if pressure is placed on the injection site immediately after injection. The use of physical modalities, including local heat as well as gentle range of motion exercises, should be introduced several days after the patient undergoes this injection technique for slipping rib syndrome. Vigorous exercises should be avoided because they will exacerbate the patient's symptomatology. Simple analgesics and nonsteroidal anti-inflammatory agents may be used concurrently with this injection technique. Laboratory evaluation for collagen vascular disease is indicated in patients suffering from costal cartilage pain in whom other joints are involved.

34

Xiphodynia

ICD-9 CODE 733.90

THE CLINICAL SYNDROME

An uncommon cause of anterior chest wall pain, xiphodynia is often misdiagnosed as pain of cardiac or upper abdominal origin. Xiphodynia syndrome is a constellation of symptoms consisting of severe intermittent anterior chest wall pain in the region of the xiphoid process that is made worse with overeating, stooping, and bending. The patient may complain of a nauseated feeling associated with the pain of xiphodynia syndrome. This xiphisternal joint appears to serve as the nidus of pain for xiphodynia syndrome.

The xiphosternal joint is often traumatized during acceleration/deceleration injuries and blunt trauma to the chest. With severe trauma, the joint may sublux or dislocate. The xiphisternal joint is also susceptible to the development of arthritis, including osteoarthritis, rheumatoid arthritis, ankylosing spondylitis, Reiter's syndrome, and psoriatic arthritis. The joint is also subject to invasion by tumor either from primary malignancies including thymoma or from metastatic disease.

SIGNS AND SYMPTOMS

Physical examination reveals that the pain of xiphodynia syndrome is reproduced with palpation or traction on the xiphoid. The xiphisternal joint may feel swollen (Fig. 34–1). Stooping or bending may reproduce the pain. Coughing may be difficult, and this may lead to inadequate pulmonary toilet in patients who have sustained trauma to the anterior chest wall. The xiphisternal joint and adjacent intercostal muscles may also be tender to palpation. The patient may also complain of a clicking sensation with movement of the joint.

TESTING

Plain radiographs are indicated in all patients who present with pain thought to be emanating from the xiphisternal joint to rule out occult bony pathology, including tumor. Based on the patient's clinical presentation, additional testing including complete blood cell count, prostate specific antigen, sedimentation rate, and antinuclear antibody testing may be indicated. Magnetic resonance imaging (MRI) of the joint is indicated if joint instability or occult mass is suspected. The following injection technique serves as both a diagnostic and therapeutic maneuver.

DIFFERENTIAL DIAGNOSIS

As with costochondritis, costosternal joint pain, devil's grip, Tietze's syndrome, and rib fractures, a significant number of patients who suffer from xiphodynia first seek medical attention because they believe they are suffering a heart attack. The patient may also believe they are suffering from ulcer or gallbladder disease. In contradistinction to most other causes of pain involving the chest wall that are musculoskeletal or neuropathic in nature, the pain of devil's grip is infectious in nature. The constitutional symptoms associated with devil's grip may lead the clinician to consider pneumonia, empyema, and, on occasion, pulmonary embolus as the most likely diagnosis.

TREATMENT

Initial treatment of xiphodynia should include a combination of simple analgesics and the nonsteroidal anti-inflammatory agents or the cyclooxygenase-2 (COX-2) inhibitors. If these medications do not adequately control the patient's symptomatology, opioid analgesics may be added during the period of acute pain.

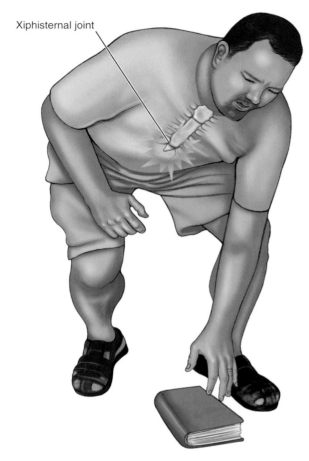

Xiphisternal joint

Figure 34–1. The xiphisternal joint is swollen in patients suffering from xiphodynia.

The local application of heat and cold may also be beneficial to provide symptomatic relief of the pain of xiphodynia. The use of an elastic rib belt may also help provide symptomatic relief in some patients. For patients who do not respond to these treatment modalities, the injection of the xiphisternal joint using a local anesthetic and steroid may be a reasonable next step.

COMPLICATIONS AND PITFALLS

The major problem in the care of patients thought to suffer from xiphodynia is the failure to identify potentially serious pathology of the thorax or upper abdomen. The major complication of injection of the xiphisternal joint is pneumothorax if the needle is placed too laterally or deeply and invades the pleural space. Infection, although rare, can occur if strict aseptic technique is not adhered to. The possibility of trauma to the contents of the mediastinum remains an ever-present possibility. This complication can be greatly decreased if the clinician plays close attention to accurate needle placement.

CLINICAL PEARLS

Patients suffering from pain emanating from the xiphisternal joint will often attribute their pain symptomatology to a heart attack or ulcer disease. Reassurance is required, although it should be remembered that this musculoskeletal pain syndrome, ulcer disease, and coronary artery disease can all coexist. The xiphoid process articulates with the sternum via the xiphisternal joint. The xiphoid process is a plate of cartilaginous bone that becomes calcified in early adulthood. The xiphisternal joint is strengthened by ligaments but can be subluxed or dislocated by blunt trauma to the anterior chest. The xiphisternal joint is innervated by the T4-7 intercostal nerves as well as the phrenic nerve. It is thought that this innervation by the phrenic nerve is responsible for the referred pain associated with xiphodynia syndrome. Tietze's syndrome, which is painful enlargement of the upper costochondral cartilage associated with viral infections, can be confused with xiphisternal syndrome, although both respond to the injection technique described.

The use of physical modalities, including local heat as well as gentle range of motion exercises, should be introduced several days after the patient undergoes this injection technique for xiphisternal joint pain. Vigorous exercises should be avoided because they will exacerbate the patient's symptomatology. Simple analgesics and nonsteroidal anti-inflammatory agents may be used concurrently with this injection technique. Laboratory evaluation for collagen vascular disease is indicated in patients suffering from xiphisternal joint pain in whom other joints are involved.

35

Winged Scapula Syndrome

ICD-9 CODE 736.89

THE CLINICAL SYNDROME

Winged scapula syndrome is an uncommon cause of musculoskeletal pain of the shoulder and posterior chest wall. Due to paralysis of the serratus anterior muscle, winged scapula syndrome begins as a painless weakness of the muscle with the resultant pathognomonic finding of winged scapula. However, due to dysfunction secondary to paralysis of the muscle, musculoskeletal pain often results. Winged scapula syndrome is often initially misdiagnosed as strain of the shoulder groups and muscles of the posterior chest wall because the onset of the syndrome often occurs after heavy exertion, most commonly after carrying heavy backpacks. The syndrome may coexist with entrapment of the suprascapular nerve.

Trauma to the long thoracic nerve of Bell is most often responsible for the development of winged scapula syndrome. Arising from the fifth, sixth, and seventh cervical nerves, the nerve is susceptible to stretch injuries and direct trauma. The nerve is often injured during first rib resection for thoracic outlet syndrome. Injuries to the brachial plexus or cervical roots may also cause scapular winging but usually in conjunction with other neurological findings.

The pain of winged scapula syndrome is aching in nature and is localized to the muscle mass of the posterior chest wall and scapula. The pain may radiate into the shoulder and upper arm. The intensity of the pain of winged scapula syndrome is mild to moderate but may produce significant functional disability that, if untreated, will continue to exacerbate the musculoskeletal component of the pain.

SIGNS AND SYMPTOMS

Regardless of the mechanism of injury to the long thoracic nerve of Bell, the common clinical feature of winged scapula syndrome is paralysis of the scapula due to weakness of the serratus anterior muscle. The pain of winged scapula syndrome generally develops after the onset of acute muscle weakness but is often erroneously attributed to overuse during vigorous exercise. On physical examination, the last 30 degrees of overhead arm extension is lost and the scapular rhythm is disrupted. By having the patient press the outstretched arms against a wall, the scapular winging is easily viewed by the clinician observing the patient from behind. The remainder of the patient's neurological examination should be within normal limits (Fig. 35–1).

TESTING

Owing to the ambiguity and confusion surrounding this clinical syndrome, testing is important to help confirm the diagnosis of winged scapula syndrome. Electromyography will help distinguish isolated damage to the long thoracic nerve of Bell associated with winged scapula syndrome from brachial plexopathy. Plain radiographs are indicated in all patients who present with winged scapula syndrome to rule out occult bony pathology. Based on the patient's clinical presentation, additional testing including complete blood cell count, uric acid, sedimentation rate, and antinuclear antibody testing may be indicated. Magnetic resonance imaging (MRI) of the brachial plexus and/or cervical spine is indicated if the patient exhibits other neurological deficits.

DIFFERENTIAL DIAGNOSIS

Lesions of the cervical spinal cord, brachial plexus, and cervical nerve roots can produce clinical symptoms that include winging of the scapula. However, such lesions should also produce additional neurological findings that will allow the clinician to distinguish these pathological conditions from the

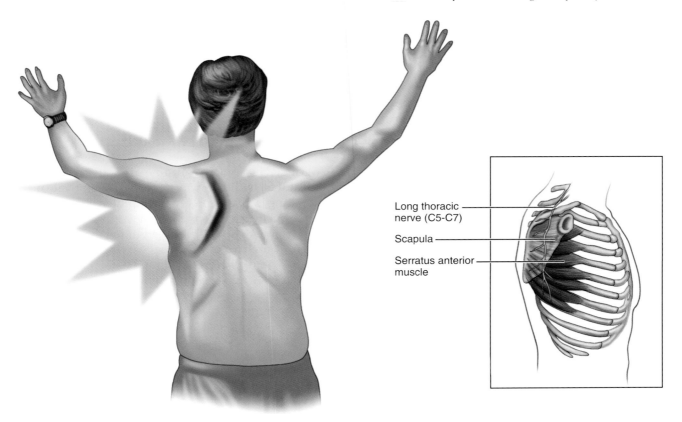

Figure 35–1. Scapular winging is best viewed by having the patient push his or her hands against the wall.

isolated neurological findings seen in winged scapula syndrome.

Pathology of the scapula or shoulder group may also confuse the clinical diagnosis.

TREATMENT

There is no specific treatment for winged scapula syndrome other than the removal of the cause of nerve entrapment, such as heavy backpacks, tumor compressing nerve, etc., and the use of an orthotic device to help stabilize the scapula to allow normal shoulder function. Initial symptomatic relief of the pain and functional disability associated with winged scapula should include a combination of the nonsteroidal anti-inflammatory agents or cyclooxygenase-2 (COX-2) inhibitors and physical therapy. The local application of heat and cold may also be beneficial. The repetitive movements or those that incite the syndrome should be avoided.

SIDE EFFECTS AND COMPLICATIONS

The major complications associated with winged scapula syndrome fall into two categories: (1)

damage to the shoulder due to the functional disability associated with the syndrome and (2) failure to recognize that the cause of winging of the scapula is the result not of an isolated lesion of the long thoracic nerve of Bell but rather a part of a larger neurological problem.

CLINICAL PEARLS

Winged scapula syndrome is a distinct clinical entity that is difficult to treat. Early removal of the offending cause of nerve entrapment should allow rapid recovery of nerve function with resultant improvement in pain and shoulder dysfunction. A careful search for other causes of winging the scapula should occur before attributing this neurological finding to winged scapula syndrome.

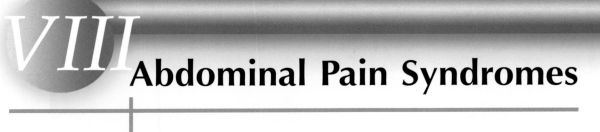

VIII Abdominal Pain Syndromes

36 Anterior Cutaneous Nerve Entrapment Syndrome

ICD-9 CODE 355.9

THE CLINICAL SYNDROME

Anterior cutaneous nerve entrapment syndrome is an uncommon cause of anterior abdominal wall pain that is a frequently overlooked clinical diagnosis. Anterior cutaneous nerve entrapment syndrome is a constellation of symptoms consisting of severe knife-like pain emanating from the anterior abdominal wall associated with the physical finding of point tenderness over the affected anterior cutaneous nerve. The pain radiates medially to the linea alba but in almost all cases does not cross the midline. Anterior cutaneous nerve entrapment syndrome occurs most commonly in young females. The patient can often localize the source of pain quite accurately by pointing to the spot at which the anterior cutaneous branch of the affected intercostal nerve pierces the fascia of the abdominal wall at the lateral border of the abdominus rectus muscle. It is at this point that anterior cutaneous branch of the intercostal nerve turns sharply in an anterior direction to provide innervation to the anterior wall. The nerve passes through a firm fibrous ring as it pierces the fascia, and it is at this point that the nerve is subject to entrapment. The nerve is accompanied through the fascia by an epigastric artery and vein. There is the potential for small amounts of abdominal fat to herniate through this fascial ring and become incarcerated, which results in further entrapment of the nerve. The pain of anterior cutaneous nerve entrapment is moderate to severe in intensity.

SIGNS AND SYMPTOMS

As mentioned, the patient can often point to the exact spot that the anterior cutaneous nerve is entrapped. Palpation of this point will often elicit sudden, sharp, lancinating pain in the distribution of the affected anterior cutaneous nerve. Voluntary contraction of the abdominal muscles will put additional pressure on the nerve and may also elicit the pain.

The patient will attempt to splint the affected nerve by keeping the thoracolumbar spine slightly flexed to avoid increasing tension on the abdominal musculature (Fig. 36–1). Having the patient do a sit-up will often reproduce the pain, as will a Valsalva maneuver.

TESTING

Plain radiographs are indicated in all patients who present with pain thought to be emanating from the lower costal cartilage and ribs to rule out occult bony pathology, including rib fracture and tumor. Radiographic evaluation of the gallbladder is indicated if cholelithiasis is suspected. Based on the patient's clinical presentation, additional testing including complete blood cell count, rectal examination with stool guaiac, sedimentation rate, and antinuclear antibody testing may be indicated. Computed tomography (CT) scan of the abdomen is indicated if intra-abdominal pathology or occult mass is suspected. Injection of the anterior cutaneous nerve at the point at which it pierces the fascia serves as both a diagnostic and therapeutic maneuver.

DIFFERENTIAL DIAGNOSIS

The differential diagnosis of anterior cutaneous nerve entrapment syndrome should consider ventral hernia, peptic ulcer disease, cholecystitis, intermittent bowel obstruction, renal calculi, angina, mesenteric vascular insufficiency, diabetic polyneuropathy, and pneumonia. Rarely, the collagen vascular diseases, including systemic lupus erythematosus and polyarteritis nodosa, may cause intermittent

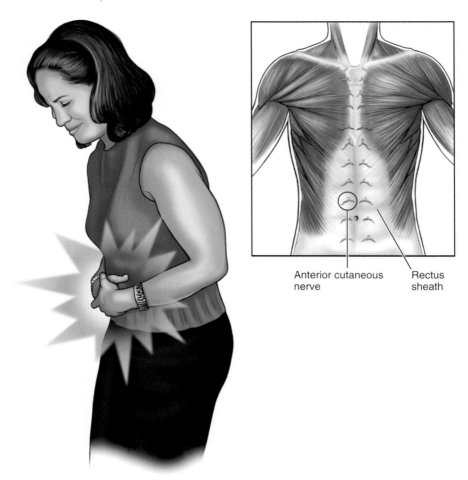

Anterior cutaneous nerve

Rectus sheath

Figure 36–1

abdominal pain as may porphyria. Because the pain of acute herpes zoster may precede the rash by 24 to 72 hours, the pain may erroneously be attributed to anterior cutaneous nerve entrapment.

TREATMENT

Initial treatment of the pain and functional disability associated with anterior cutaneous entrapment syndrome should include a combination of the nonsteroidal anti-inflammatory agents or the cyclooxygenase-2 (COX-2) inhibitors and physical therapy. The local application of heat and cold may also be beneficial. The repetitive movements that incite the syndrome should be avoided. For patients who do not respond to these treatment modalities, injection of the anterior cutaneous nerve at the point at which the nerve pierces the fascia with a local anesthetic and steroid may be a reasonable next step. If the symptoms of anterior cutaneous entrapment syndrome persist, surgical exploration and decompression of the anterior cutaneous nerve are indicated.

SIDE EFFECTS AND COMPLICATIONS

The major complications associated with anterior cutaneous entrapment syndrome fall into two categories: (1) iatrogenically induced complications due to incorrect diagnosis and (2) failure of the clinician to recognize that a hernia coexists with the nerve entrapment until bowel ischemia occurs.

CLINICAL PEARLS

Patients suffering from pain emanating from anterior cutaneous nerve entrapment syndrome often attribute their pain symptomatology to a gallbladder attack or ulcer disease. Reassurance is required, although it should be remembered that this musculoskeletal pain syndromes and intra-abdominal pathology can coexist. The use of physical modalities, including local heat as well as gentle range of motion exercises, should be introduced several days after the patient undergoes this injection technique for anterior cutaneous nerve entrapment syndrome. Vigorous exercises should be avoided because they will exacerbate the patient's symptomatology. Simple analgesics and nonsteroidal anti-inflammatory agents may be used concurrently with the abovementioned injection technique. Radiographic evaluation for intra-abdominal pathology is indicated in patients suffering from anterior abdominal pain of unclear etiology.

37 Acute Intermittent Porphyria

ICD-9 CODE 277.1

THE CLINICAL SYNDROME

Acute intermittent porphyria is an uncommon cause of abdominal pain that frequently confounds the diagnostic efforts of even the most astute clinician. The porphyrias are disorders of heme synthesis that can produce a wide range of clinical symptomatology. There are a number of different types of porphyrias, each of which presents in a distinct clinical manner that reflects the specific enzyme deficiency of the heme biosynthetic pathway. The porphyrias can be either inherited or acquired. The main clinical manifestations of the porphyrias are neurological dysfunction and the unique clinical finding of cutaneous sensitivity to sunlight.

Acute intermittent porphyria is an autosomal dominant trait with variable clinical expression. The incidence of the gene responsible for acute intermittent porphyria is thought to be 1 in 100,000 individuals. The disease rarely manifests itself before puberty. Acute abdominal pain is usually the first clinical expression of the disease. As the name implies, the pain of acute intermittent porphyria is intermittent and colicky in nature. The pain may be localized to the abdomen or may radiate to the flanks. The patient may also exhibit neurological symptoms suggesting dysfunction of both the central and peripheral nervous systems. Port wine urine, which is characteristic of the hepatic porphyrias, including acute intermittent porphyria, is often seen during acute attacks.

SIGNS AND SYMPTOMS

Although the complaints of abdominal pain are often quite impressive in patients suffering from acute intermittent porphyria, the abdominal examination is often bland (Fig. 37–1). Vomiting occasionally occurs. Tachycardia and autonomic dysfunction including sweating are common, as is labile hypertension. Occasionally, urinary retention may occur and may confuse the clinical diagnosis, especially if port wine urine is present. Neurological findings including attenuated deep tendon reflexes and decreased distal sensation suggestive of peripheral neuropathy are often present. Cranial nerve involvement is less common, but can be severe. Mental disturbance ranging from agitation to frank psychosis can occur in up to one third of patients with acute intermittent porphyria. A substrate of nervousness and anxiety often makes the care of these patients difficult. Alcohol, pregnancy, barbiturates, and oral contraceptives may precipitate attacks of acute intermittent porphyria.

TESTING

Given the usual delay in the diagnosis of acute intermittent porphyria, there usually is no shortage of testing being done. Unfortunately, most standard laboratory testing will not point the clinician toward a diagnosis of acute intermittent porphyria. Specifically, liver function tests are normal. A mild normocytic, normochromic anemia is sometimes present. Freshly passed urine is colorless but will turn to a port wine color if exposed to light. Given the low incidence of porphyria, qualitative urine screening tests such as the Watson-Schwartz test is a reasonable first step in diagnosing porphyria. If positive, quantitative testing such as gas chromatographic measurements for amino-levulinic acid should be performed.

DIFFERENTIAL DIAGNOSIS

Essentially all causes of acute intermittent abdominal pain must be included in the differential diagnosis. It is important that the clinician take a careful history and perform a careful physical examination to rule out life-threatening causes of acute, intermit-

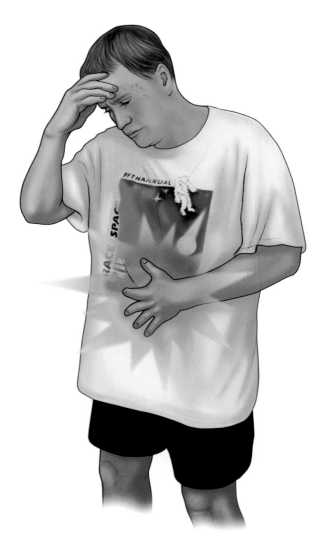

Figure 37–1

in patients suffering from acute intermittent porphyria, psychogenic causes of abdominal pain must be included in the differential diagnosis.

TREATMENT

Acute attacks of acute intermittent porphyria can be aborted by the intravenous administration of large quantities of carbohydrates such as glucose. Hematin can also be given intravenously and is seemingly well tolerated. Avoidance of barbiturates, anticonvulsants, and alcohol is imperative to avoid exacerbating the symptoms of acute attacks of acute intermittent porphyria. Careful attention to fluid and electrolyte balance is also important. Despite careful treatment, fatalities during acute attacks are not unheard of.

COMPLICATIONS AND SIDE EFFECTS

The major complications surrounding acute intermittent porphyria relate to misdiagnosis and failure to correct metabolic and electrolyte abnormalities during acute attacks. Barbiturates and anticonvulsants are often erroneously given to control seizures associated with acute intermittent porphyria, which only worsen the porphyria, creating a vicious negative feedback cycle that may ultimately kill the patient.

CLINICAL PEARLS

The cause of abdominal pain in acute intermittent porphyria is thought to be the result of intermittent autonomic dysfunction causing abnormal gut motility with alternating spasm and obstruction. The incidence of psychiatric abnormalities in patients suffering from acute intermittent porphyria often confounds the clinician and complicates treatment. It has been said that to make the diagnosis, the clinician must think of it first. Nowhere is this statement more true than in the case of acute intermittent porphyria.

tent abdominal pain, such as ischemic bowel, volvulus, acute appendicitis, etc. The key distinguishing factor in acute intermittent porphyria is that the patient's complaints of severe abdominal pain and their benign abdominal examination do not correlate. Given the high incidence of psychiatric abnormalities

38 *Radiation Enteritis*

THE CLINICAL SYNDROME

As cancer patients live longer, clinicians are being called on with greater frequency to manage the side effects and complications of cancer therapy. One such complication is radiation enteritis. This complication of radiation therapy can occur after radiation to the abdomen or pelvis. Early symptoms of radiation enteritis are due to mucosal edema and ulceration and include abdominal pain, nausea, and vomiting, as well as a sensation of needing to move one's bowels and/or tenesmus. Late symptoms that are more related to radiation-induced scarring and narrowing of the bowel include small-caliber stools, rectal burning, and mucoid stools. The intensity of pain is mild to moderate and cramping in character. The onset of the early symptoms of radiation enteritis can begin within 1 week to 10 days after the completion of radiation therapy, and the late symptoms can occur months to years later.

SIGNS AND SYMPTOMS

Physical examination of the patient suffering from radiation enteritis will reveal diffuse abdominal tenderness and hyperactive bowel sounds. Mild abdominal distension may be present. Signs of acute peritoneal irritation suggestive of perforated viscus, such as rebound tenderness, are absent. The patient may exhibit frequent defecation of mucoid stools, diarrhea, and vomiting.

The patient will appear systemically ill but not septic (Fig. 38–1).

TESTING

Colonoscopy provides the clinician with definitive evidence or radiation enteritis while at the same time helping to exclude other causes of abdominal pain that may mimic this clinical syndrome. Based on the patient's clinical presentation, additional testing including complete blood cell count, sedimentation rate, and stool and blood cultures for infectious enteritis may be indicated. Computed tomography (CT) scan of the abdomen with oral and intravenous contrast is indicated if occult mass or abscess is suspected.

DIFFERENTIAL DIAGNOSIS

The history of previous radiation therapy is necessary to consider the diagnosis of radiation enteritis. Unfortunately, the very problem that necessitated radiation therapy in the first place, malignancy, can recur and produce clinical symptomatology indistinguishable from that of radiation enteritis. Given the immunocompromised state of most patients who have received radiation therapy, the possibility of infectious enteritis or intra-abdominal abscess must always be included in the differential diagnosis. It must be remembered that other causes of abdominal pain, including diverticulitis, bowel obstruction, and appendicitis, may also occur in conjunction with radiation enteritis.

TREATMENT

Symptom management is the primary thrust of the treatment of radiation enteritis. Careful attention to the patient's fluid and metabolic status during the acute phases of the disease is crucial to avoid complications. Psyllium will help the patient with diarrhea and with mucoid stools and may decrease the sensations of needing to frequently move the bowels. Anticholinergics such as dicyclomine and antiperistaltics such as loperamide can help decrease diarrhea. Zinc oxide ointment and sitz baths with aluminum acetate soaks will help with the symptoms of tenesmus and rectal pain. Steroid and sucralfate

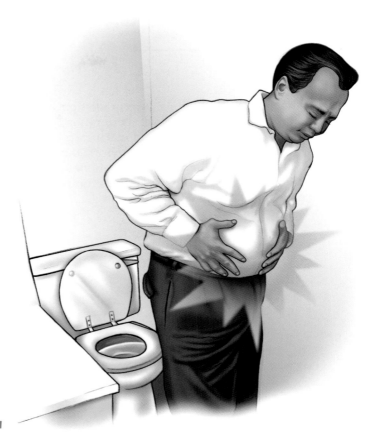

Figure 38–1

enemas have also been reported to provide symptomatic relief in difficult cases of radiation enteritis.

SIDE EFFECTS AND COMPLICATIONS

The potential for complications after radiation therapy is high. Spontaneous bowel perforation, stenosis, fistula formation, bleeding, and malabsorption occur with sufficient frequency to complicate the management of this painful condition. As mentioned, the potential for recurrence of tumor and infectious complications remains ever present.

CLINICAL PEARLS

The treatment of the symptoms associated with radiation enteritis should be part of the overall management of the patient with cancer. The recognition and treatment of symptoms other than pain are often delayed while the clinician focuses on pain control, further compounding the patient's suffering. Vigilance for life-threatening complications of radiation enteritis, including bowel perforation, is mandatory to avoid disaster.

39

Liver Pain

ICD-9 CODE 573.8

THE CLINICAL SYNDROME

Liver pain is a common clinical occurrence, but it is often poorly diagnosed and treated. The liver can serve as a source of pain in and of itself via the sympathetic nervous system and via referred pain secondary to peritoneal irritation via the intercostal and subcostal nerves. Pain that emanates from the liver itself tends to be ill defined and may be referred primarily to the epigastrium. It is dull and aching in character and is mild to moderate in severity. It can be related to swelling of the liver and concomitant stretching of the liver capsule or due to distention of the veins as is seen with portal obstruction. This pain is carried via sympathetic fibers from the celiac ganglion that enter the liver along with the hepatic artery and vein. This type of liver pain responds poorly to adjuvant analgesics. Occasionally, hepatic enlargement will cause diaphragmatic irritation, which will produce pain that is referred to the supraclavicular region. This referred pain is transmitted via the phrenic nerve and is often misdiagnosed.

Referred liver pain is caused by mechanical irritation and inflammation of the inferior pleura and peritoneum. This pain is somatic in nature and is carried primarily via the lower intercostal and subcostal nerves. This somatic pain is sharp and pleuritic in nature and is moderate to severe in intensity. This pain responds more favorably to nonsteroidal anti-inflammatory agents and opioid analgesics compared with sympathetically mediated liver pain.

SIGNS AND SYMPTOMS

The clinical presentation of liver pain will be directly related to whether the pain is mediated via the sympathetic or somatic nervous system or both. In patients with sympathetically mediated pain, the abdominal examination may reveal hepatomegaly with tenderness to palpation of the liver. Primary tumor or metastatic disease may also be identified. The remainder of the abdominal examination will be bland. Auscultation over the liver will fail to reveal a friction rub in most cases. As mentioned, the patient may complain of ill-defined pain in the supraclavicular region (Fig. 39–1).

Patients with somatically mediated liver pain will present in an entirely different manner. The patient will often splint the right lower chest wall and abdomen and take small, short breaths to avoid exacerbating the pain. The patient may avoid coughing because of the pain and accumulated upper airway secretions, and atelectasis may be a problem. The abdominal examination may reveal signs of peritoneal irritation over the right upper quadrant. A friction rub is often present with auscultation over the liver. The liver may be extremely tender to palpation. Primary tumor and/or metastatic disease may be present.

TESTING

Testing for patients with liver pain should be aimed at identifying the primary source of liver disease responsible for the pain as well as ruling out other pathological processes that may be responsible for the pain. Plain radiographs of the chest and abdomen, including an upright abdominal film, are indicated in all patients who present with pain thought to be emanating from the liver. Radiographs of the ribs are indicated to rule out occult bony pathology, including tumor. Based on the patient's clinical presentation, additional testing including complete blood cell count, automated chemistries, liver function test, sedimentation rate, and antinuclear antibody testing may be indicated. Computed tomography (CT) scan of the lower thoracic

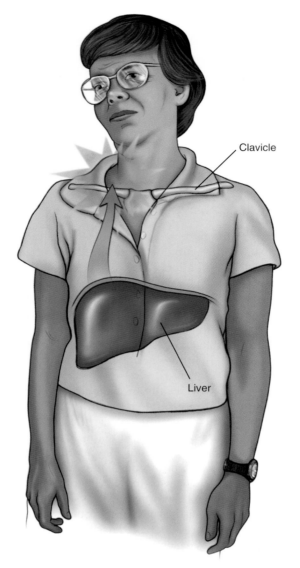

Figure 39–1

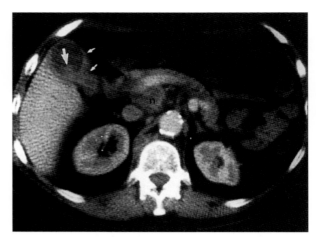

Figure 39–2. Gallbladder carcinoma (*small arrows*) presenting as thickening of the gallbladder wall with a gallstone (*large arrow*) and metastasis to lymph nodes (*n*). (From Haaga, JR, Lanzieri CF, Sartoris UJ, Zerhouni EA: Computed Tomography and Magnetic Resonance Imaging of the Whole Body, 3rd ed. St Louis, Mosby, 1994.)

contents and abdomen is indicated in most patients suffering from liver pain to rule out occult pulmonary and intra-abdominal pathology, including cancer of the gallbladder and pancreas (Fig. 39–2). Differential neural blockade on an anatomic basis can serve as both a diagnostic and therapeutic maneuver (see Treatment).

DIFFERENTIAL DIAGNOSIS

Pain of hepatic origin must be taken seriously. It is often the result of an underlying serious disease, such as biliary malignancy, portal hypertension, hepatic metastatic disease, etc. Pain emanating from the liver is often mistaken for pain of cardiac or gallbladder origin and can lead to visits to the emergency depart-

ment and unnecessary cardiac and gastrointestinal work-ups. If trauma has occurred, liver pain may coexist with fractured ribs or fractures of the sternum itself that can be missed on plain radiographs and may require radionucleotide bone scanning for proper identification.

Neuropathic pain involving the chest wall may also be confused or coexist with liver pain. Examples of such neuropathic pain include diabetic polyneuropathies and acute herpes zoster involving the lower thoracic and upper lumbar nerves. The possibility of diseases of the structures of the inferior mediastinum and retroperitoneum remains ever present and at times can be difficult to diagnose. Pathological processes that inflame the pleura, such as pulmonary embolus, infection, and Borneholm's disease, may also mimic or coexist with pain of hepatic origin.

TREATMENT

Initial treatment of liver pain should include a combination of simple analgesics and the nonsteroidal anti-inflammatory agents or the cyclooxygenase-2 (COX-2) inhibitors. If these medications do not adequately control the patient's symptomatology, an opioid analgesic may be added.

The local application of heat and cold may also be beneficial to provide symptomatic relief of liver pain. The use of an elastic rib belt over the liver may also help provide symptomatic relief. For patients who do not respond to these treatment modalities, an intercostal nerve block using a local anesthetic and steroid may be a reasonable next step. If the pain is thought to be sympathetically mediated, a celiac plexus block is a reasonable next step. This technique provides both diagnostic and therapeutic benefit. If the pain is thought to be somatic in nature, intercostal nerve blocks should be the next step. It should be remembered that pain of hepatic origin may be both somatic and sympathetic in nature and require both celiac plexus and intercostal nerve block for complete control.

COMPLICATIONS AND PITFALLS

The major problem in the care of patients thought to suffer from liver pain is the failure to identify potentially serious pathology of the thorax or upper abdomen. Given the proximity of the pleural space, pneumothorax after intercostal nerve block is a distinct possibility. The incidence of the complication is less than 1%, but it occurs with greater frequency in patients with chronic obstructive pulmonary disease. Although uncommon, infection including liver abscess remains an ever-present possibility, especially in the immunocompromised patient with cancer. Early detection of infection is crucial to avoid potentially life-threatening sequelae.

CLINICAL PEARLS

Liver pain is often poorly diagnosed and treated. Correct diagnosis as to the cause of liver pain and as to the nerves subserving the pain is necessary to properly treat this painful condition and to avoid overlooking serious intrathoracic or intra-abdominal pathology. Intercostal nerve block is a simple technique that can produce dramatic relief for patients suffering from liver pain thought to be somatically mediated. Celiac plexus block is technically more demanding and should be performed only by those well versed in the technique and potential complications.

40 Abdominal Angina

ICD-9 CODE 557.1

THE CLINICAL SYNDROME

Abdominal angina is an uncommon cause of intermittent abdominal pain. Patients suffering from abdominal angina complain of severe cramping abdominal pain that begins 15 to 30 minutes after eating (Figs. 40–1 and 40–2). This postprandial pain persists for 2 to 3 hours. Additional ingestion of food aggravates the patient's pain, thus forcing the patient to stop eating. Weight loss is common. As the disease progresses, malabsorption and diarrhea occur due to mucosal and mural injury, which further exacerbates the patient's weight loss.

The cause of abdominal angina is arterial vascular insufficiency. The term *angina* is used because the pain occurs only after eating, when the insufficient fixed arterial supply is unable to meet the increased demands needed to support digestion. The most common cause of abdominal angina is stenosis of the celiac artery with inadequate collateralization. Aneurysms of the superior mesenteric artery, the vasculitides, fibromuscular hyperplasia, and tumor encroachment on the celiac artery have also been implicated as causes of abdominal angina.

SIGNS AND SYMPTOMS

Physical examination of the patient suffering from abdominal angina will reveal diffuse abdominal tenderness. Mild abdominal distension may be present. Signs of acute peritoneal irritation suggestive of perforated viscus, such as rebound tenderness, are absent. The patient may exhibit frequent defecation of mucoid stools, diarrhea, and vomiting. The patient appears systemically ill but not septic.

TESTING

The diagnosis of abdominal angina is based on clinical history. Angiography of the celiac artery provides the clinician with proof of vascular insufficiency and often provides the etiology of the problem. Barium enema demonstrates the classic finding of thumbprinting that is strongly suggestive of mucosal ischemia (Fig. 40–3). Colonoscopy reveals localized hemorrhage and ulceration of the affected mucosa. Based on the patient's clinical presentation, additional testing including complete blood cell count, sedimentation rate, and stool and blood cultures for infectious enteritis may be indicated. Given the possibility that the patient's abdominal angina is due to vasculitis, a collagen vascular work-up is indicated in all patients suffering from abdominal angina. Computed tomography (CT) scan of the abdomen with oral and intravenous contrast is indicated if occult mass or abscess is suspected.

DIFFERENTIAL DIAGNOSIS

Any disease process that can produce ischemic bowel can mimic the pain of abdominal angina. The vasculitides, including polyarteritis nodosum and Henoch-Schönlein purpura, can also cause the symptoms of abdominal angina. Embolic disease that may cause occlusion of the vascular supply to the gut should also be considered. The possibility of infectious enteritis must always be included in the differential diagnosis. It must be remembered that other causes of abdominal pain, including diverticulitis, bowel obstruction, and appendicitis, may also occur in conjunction with abdominal angina.

TREATMENT

The only definitive treatment of abdominal angina is correction of the arterial insufficiency via either

146

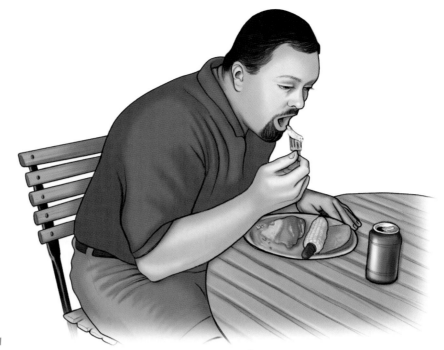

Figure 40–1

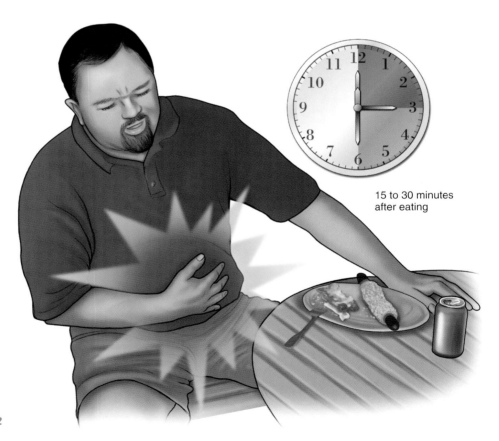

15 to 30 minutes
after eating

Figure 40–2

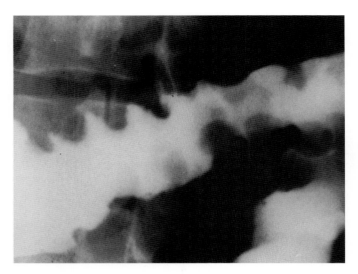

Figure 40–3. Thumbprinting in acute ischemic colitis at the splenic flexure. (From Grainger RG, Allison D: Grainger & Allison's Diagnostic Radiology: A Textbook of Medical Imaging, 3rd ed. New York, Churchill Livingstone, 1997, p 1036.)

angioplasty or surgical revascularization. Careful attention to the patient's fluid and metabolic status is crucial to avoid complications. Anticholinergics such as dicyclomine and antiperistaltics such as loperamide can help decrease diarrhea. Small, frequent feedings may also help palliate the postprandial pain.

SIDE EFFECTS AND COMPLICATIONS

The potential for complications in patients suffering from abdominal angina is high. Spontaneous bowel perforation, stenosis, fistula formation, bleeding, and malabsorption occur with sufficient frequency to complicate the management of this painful condition. Untreated, abdominal angina frequently progresses to bowel infarction.

CLINICAL PEARLS

The treatment of the symptoms associated with abdominal angina is difficult, and ultimately, correction of the vascular insufficiency will be required. Vigilance for life-threatening complications of abdominal angina, including bowel infarction, is mandatory to avoid disaster.

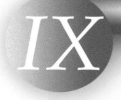

IX

Lumbar Spine Pain

41

Epidural Abscess

ICD-9 CODE 324.1

THE CLINICAL SYNDROME

Epidural abscess is an uncommon cause of spine pain that, if undiagnosed, can result in paralysis and/or life-threatening complications. Epidural abscess can occur anywhere in the spine as well as intracranially. It can occur spontaneously via hematogenous seeding, most frequently as a result of urinary tract infections that spread to the spinal epidural space via Batson's plexus. More commonly, epidural abscess occurs after instrumentation of the spine including surgery and epidural nerve blocks. The literature has suggested that the administration of steroids into the epidural space results in immuno-suppression with a resultant increase in the incidence of epidural abscess. Although theoretically plausible, the statistical evidence given the thousands of epidural steroid injections performed around the country on a daily basis calls this belief into question.

The patient with epidural abscess initially presents with ill-defined pain in the segment of the spine affected (e.g., cervical, thoracic, or lumbar) (Fig. 41–1). This pain will become more intense and localized as the abscess increases in size and compresses neural structures. Low-grade fever and vague constitutional symptoms including malaise and anorexia will progress to frank sepsis with a high-grade fever, rigors, and chills. At this point, the patient will begin to experience sensory and motor deficits as well as bowel and bladder symptomatology as the result of neural compromise. As the abscess continues to expand, compromise of the vascular supply to the affected spinal cord and nerve will occur with resultant ischemia and, if untreated, infarction and permanent neurological deficits.

SIGNS AND SYMPTOMS

The patient with epidural abscess initially presents with ill-defined pain in the general area of the infection. At this point, there may be mild pain on range of motion of the affected segments. The neurological examination will be within normal limits. A low-grade fever and/or night sweats may be present. Theoretically, if the patient has received steroids, these constitutional symptoms may be attenuated or their onset delayed. As the abscess increases in size, the patient will appear acutely ill with fever, rigors, and chills. The clinician may be able to identify neurological findings suggestive of spinal nerve root and/or spinal cord compression. Subtle findings that point toward the development of myelopathy (e.g., Babinski's sign, clonus, and decreased perineal sensation) may be overlooked if not carefully sought out. As compression of the involved neural structures continues, the patient's neurological status may deteriorate quite rapidly. If diagnosis is not made, irreversible motor and sensory deficit will result.

TESTING

Myelography is still considered the best test to ascertain compromise of the spinal cord and exiting nerve roots by an extrinsic mass such as an epidural abscess. However, in this era of readily available magnetic resonance imaging (MRI) and high-speed computed tomography (CT) scanning, it may be more prudent to obtain this noninvasive testing first rather than wait for a radiologist or spine surgeon to perform a myelogram (Fig. 41–2). Both MRI and CT are highly accurate in the diagnosis of epidural abscess and are probably more accurate than myelography in the diagnosis of intrinsic disease of the spinal cord, spinal tumor, etc. All patients suspected of suffering from epidural abscess should undergo laboratory testing consisting of complete blood cell count, sedimentation rate, and automated blood

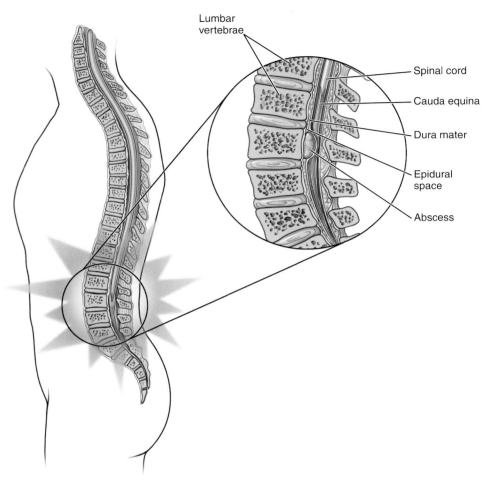

Figure 41–1

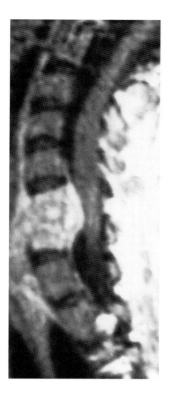

Figure 41–2. Osteomyelitis, C6-7 diskitis, and epidural abscess. After administration of Gd-DTPA, there is diffuse enhancement of the vertebral bodies and epidural abscess (SE 500/15 with Gd-DTPA). (From Stark DD, Bradley WG Jr: Magnetic Resonance Imaging, 3rd ed. St Louis, Mosby, 1999, p 1846.)

Table 41–1. Algorithm for Spinal Cord Compression Due to Epidural Abscess

• Obtain stat blood and urine cultures.
• Immediately start high-dose antibiotics that cover *Staphylococcus aureus.*
• Immediately obtain the most readily available spinal imaging technique that can confirm the presence of spinal cord compression, such as abscess, tumor, and others.
    Computed tomography
    Magnetic resonance imaging
    Myelography
• Simultaneously obtain emergency consultation from a spinal surgeon.
• Continuously and carefully monitor the patient's neurological status.
• If any of the above are unavailable, arrange emergency transfer of the patient to a tertiary care center via the most rapidly available transportation.
• Repeat imaging and obtain a repeat surgical consultation if there is any deterioration in the patient's neurological status.

chemistries. Blood and urine cultures should be immediately obtained in all patients thought to be suffering from epidural abscess to allow immediate implementation of antibiotic therapy while the work-up is in progress. Gram stains and cultures of the abscess material should also be obtained, but antibiotic treatment should not be delayed waiting for this information.

TREATMENT

The rapid initiation of treatment of epidural abscess is mandatory if the patient is to avoid the sequelae of permanent neurological deficit or death. The treatment of epidural abscess is aimed at two goals: (1) treatment of the infection with antibiotics and (2) drainage of the abscess to relieve compression on neural structures. Because the vast majority of epidural abscesses are caused by *Staphylococcus aureus,* antibiotics such as vancomycin that will treat staphylococcal infection should be started immediately after blood and urine culture samples are taken. Antibiotic therapy can be tailored to the culture and sensitivity reports as they become available. As men-

tioned, antibiotic therapy should not be delayed while waiting for definitive diagnosis if epidural abscess is being considered as part of the differential diagnosis.

Antibiotics alone will rarely successfully treat an epidural abscess unless the diagnosis is made very early in the course of the disease; thus, drainage of the abscess will be required to affect full recovery. Drainage of the epidural abscess is usually accomplished via decompression laminectomy and evacuation of the abscess. More recently, interventional radiologists have been successful in draining epidural abscesses percutaneously using drainage catheters placed with the use of CT or MRI guidance. Serial CT or MRI scans are useful in following the resolution of epidural abscess and should be repeated immediately at the first sign of negative change in the patient's neurological status.

DIFFERENTIAL DIAGNOSIS

The diagnosis of epidural abscess should be strongly considered in any patient with spine pain and fever, especially if the patient has undergone spinal instrumentation or epidural nerve blocks for either surgical anesthesia or pain control. Other pathological processes that must be considered in the differential diagnosis include intrinsic disease of the spinal cord, such as demyelinating disease and syringomyelia, as well as other processes that can result in compression of the spinal cord and exiting nerve roots, such as metastatic tumor, Paget's disease, and neurofibromatosis. As a general rule, unless the patient has concomitant infection, none of these diseases will routinely be associated with fever, just with back pain.

SIDE EFFECTS AND COMPLICATIONS

Failure to rapidly and accurately diagnosis and treat epidural abscess can only result in disaster for the clinician and patient alike. The insidious onset of neurological deficit associated with epidural abscess can lull the clinician into a sense of false security that can result in permanent neurological damage. If epidural abscess or other causes of spinal cord compression are suspected, the algorithm listed in Table 41–1 should be followed.

CLINICAL PEARLS

Delay in diagnosis puts the patient and clinician at tremendous risk for a poor outcome. The clinician should assume that all patients who present with fever and back pain have an epidural abscess until proved otherwise and should treat accordingly. Over-reliance on a single negative or equivocal imaging test is a mistake. Serial CT or MRI testing is indicated should there be any deterioration in the patient's neurological status.

42 Multiple Myeloma

ICD-9 CODE 203.0

THE CLINICAL SYNDROME

Multiple myeloma is an uncommon cause of back pain that is frequently initially misdiagnosed. It is a unique disease in that it may cause pain via several mechanisms that can act either alone or in concert. These mechanisms include invasion or compression of pain-sensitive structures (1) by the tumor itself, (2) by the products that the tumor produces, and (3) by the host response to the tumor and its products.

Although the exact etiology of multiple myeloma is unknown, the following facts have been elucidated. There appears to be a genetic predisposition to the development of myeloma. It is also known that exposure to radiation increases the incidence of the disease, as witnessed in survivors of the nuclear bombs used in World War II. RNA viruses have also been implicated in the evolution of multiple myeloma. The disease is rare under 40 years of age, with a median age of diagnosis of 60. There is a gender predilection to males. Blacks have twice the incidence of multiple myeloma compared with whites. Worldwide, the incidence of multiple myeloma is 3 per 100,000 population.

The most common clinical presentation of multiple myeloma is back and rib pain. It occurs in more than 70% of patients ultimately diagnosed with the disease. These bone lesions are osteolytic in nature and are best diagnosed with plain radiography rather than with radionucleotide bone scanning. Pain with movement is common, and hypercalcemia occurs with sufficient frequency to be the presenting symptom in many patients suffering from multiple myeloma. Life-threatening infection, anemia, bleeding, and renal failure are often present in conjunction with the symptoms of pain. Hyperviscosity of the serum that is the result of the products of tumor production may lead to cerebrovascular accidents.

SIGNS AND SYMPTOMS

Pain is the most common clinical complaint that will ultimately lead the clinician to the diagnosis of multiple myeloma (Fig. 42–1). Seemingly minor trauma may cause pathological vertebral compression or rib fractures. Pain on movement of the affected bones is a common finding on physical examination, as is the finding of tumor mass on palpation of the skull and other affected bones. Neurological findings either based on neural compression secondary to tumor or fracture or as a result of cerebrovascular accident are often present. A positive Trousseau's and Chvostek's sign due to hypercalcemia may also be elicited. Anasarca due to renal failure, if present, is an ominous prognostic sign.

TESTING

The presence of Bence Jones protein in the urine, anemia, and increased M protein on serum protein electrophoresis point strongly to the diagnosis of multiple myeloma. Classic punched-out bone lesions in the skull and spine on plain radiographs are pathognomonic for the disease (Fig. 42–2). Because there is little osteoclastic activity present in patients suffering from multiple myeloma, radionucleotide bone scanning can be amazingly negative in the face of diffuse bony destruction. Magnetic resonance imaging (MRI) is indicated in any patient thought to be suffering from multiple myeloma who exhibits signs of spinal cord compression. Serum creatine testing as well as automated blood chemistries that include serum calcium determinations are indicated in all patients with multiple myeloma.

DIFFERENTIAL DIAGNOSIS

A variety of other abnormalities of the bone marrow, including the heavy chain diseases and

155

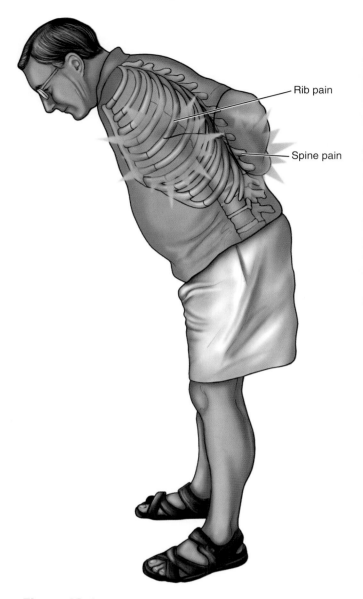

Figure 42–1

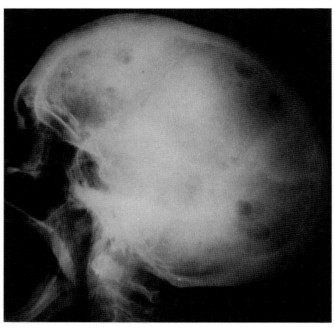

Figure 42–2. Myelomatosis. Well-defined "punched-out" lesions are shown in the calvaria. (From Grainger RG, Allison D: Grainger & Allison's Diagnostic Radiology: A Textbook of Medical Imaging, 3rd ed. New York, Churchill Livingstone, 1997, p 1704.)

Waldenström's macroglobulinemia, can mimic the clinical presentation of multiple myeloma. Amyloidosis also shares a number of common clinical signs and symptoms. Metastatic disease from prostate and breast cancer can also produce pathological fractures of the spine and ribs as well as calvarial metastases that may be mistaken for multiple myeloma. It should be remembered that there is a small group of patients who suffer from benign monoclonal gammopathy, which in most patients requires no therapy but can mimic the laboratory findings of multiple myeloma.

TREATMENT

Treatment of multiple myeloma is aimed at the treatment of progressive bone lesions and the reduction in serum myeloma proteins. Both of these goals are accomplished with the use of radiation therapy and chemotherapy either alone or in combination. High-dose pulsed steroids have also been shown to provide symptomatic relief and to extend life expectancy in patients suffering from multiple myeloma.

Initial treatment of the pain associated with multiple myeloma should include a combination of the nonsteroidal anti-inflammatory agents or cyclooxygenase-2 (COX-2) inhibitors. The addition of opioid analgesics may be required to control the more severe pain of pathological fractures. Orthotic devices such as the Cash brace and rib belts may help stabilize the spine and ribs and should be considered if there are pathological fractures. The local application of heat and cold may also be beneficial. The repetitive movements that incite the syndrome should be avoided. For patients who do not respond to these treatment modalities, the injection of the affected areas with a local anesthetic and steroid using either intercostal or epidural nerve blocks is a reasonable next step. The spinal administration of opioids may also be benefi-

46 *Ankylosing Spondylitis*

THE CLINICAL SYNDROME

Ankylosing spondylitis is an inflammatory disease of the spine, sacroiliac joints, and occasionally the extra-articular structures including the eye. It is also known as *Marie-Strumpell disease*. The etiology of ankylosing spondylitis is unknown, but autoimmune-mediated mechanisms have been implicated. Approximately 90% of patients suffering from ankylosing spondylitis have the histocompatibility antigen HLA B-27 compared with 7% of the general population. The significance of this fact is unknown but provides the basis for a diagnostic test to aid in the diagnosis of the disease. Ankylosing spondylitis occurs three times more frequently in men, and symptoms usually appear by the third decade of life. Onset of the disease after the age of 40 is rare.

Sacroiliitis is often one of the earliest manifestations of ankylosing spondylitis. This finding usually presents as morning stiffness and a deep aching pain of insidious onset in the low back and over the sacroiliac joints. This stiffness improves with activity and then reappears with periods if inactive. The pain will worsen as the disease progresses, and nocturnal exacerbations with significant sleep disturbance are common. Tenderness over the spine, sacroiliac joints, costosternal junction, and greater trochanters are common. Pain and stiffness of the peripheral joints including the hips and shoulders are present in 30% to 40% of patients suffering from ankylosing spondylitis. The character of the pain of ankylosing spondylitis is dull and aching, and its intensity is mild to moderate. Occasionally, acute uveitis can occur, as can aortic valvular disease.

SIGNS AND SYMPTOMS

Clinically, the patient with ankylosing spondylitis will complain of back and sacroiliac pain and stiffness that is worse in the morning and after periods of prolonged activity (Fig. 46–1). The patient may complain of a limitation of range of motion of the lateral spine and, on occasion, chest expansion. This limitation of range of motion is due to a combination of bony ankylosis and muscle spasm that the clinician may be able to identify on physical examination. Tenderness to palpation of the iliac crests, greater trochanter, and axial skeleton is a common finding in ankylosing spondylitis. As the disease progresses, the lumbar lordosis disappears and atrophy of the gluteal muscles may occur. A thoracic kyphosis develops, and the neck is forward flexed. Hip ankylosis may occur with hip involvement, and the patient will often compensate with flexion at the knee. Spinal fracture with resultant spinal cord injury may occur due to the rigid and inflexible nature of the spine. Anterior uveitis will present with photophobia, decreased visual acuity, and excessive lacrimation and represents an ophthalmological emergency.

TESTING

Plain radiographs of the sacroiliac joints will usually allow the clinician to diagnose ankylosing spondylitis. Erosion of the sacroiliac joints produces a characteristic symmetrical "pseudowidening" that is diagnostic of the disease (Fig. 46–2). Magnetic resonance imaging (MRI) of the spine provides the clinician with the best information regarding the contents of the lumbar spine. MRI is highly accurate and helps to identify abnormalities that may put the patient at risk for the development of myelopathy. In patients who cannot undergo MRI, such as a patient with a pacemaker, computed tomography (CT) or myelography is a reasonable second choice.

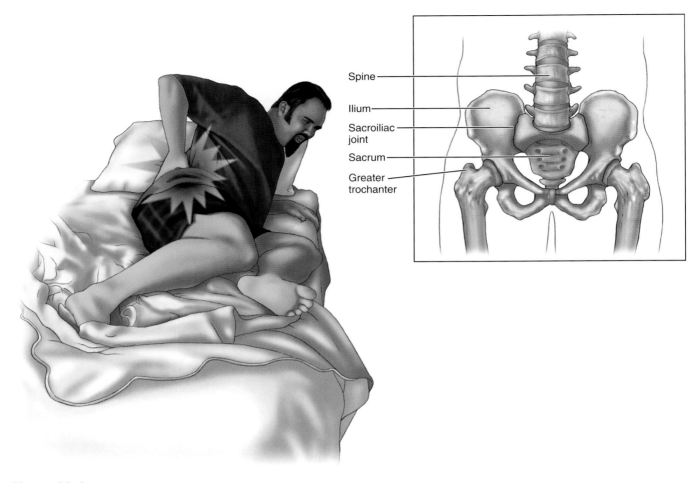

Figure 46–1

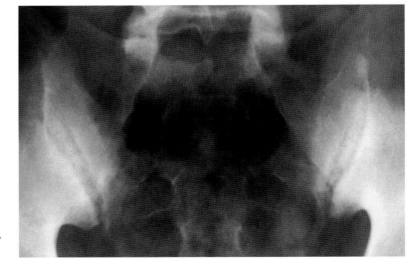

Figure 46–2. Anteroposterior Ferguson view of the sacroiliac joints in a patient with ankylosing spondylitis. There is bilateral symmetrical involvement. There are small, succinct erosions involving both sides of the joint, with limited bone repair. (From Brower AC: Disorders of the sacroiliac joint. Radiology 1978;1:3.)

Radionucleotide bone scanning and plain radiography are indicated if fracture or bony abnormality such as metastatic disease is being considered in the differential diagnosis.

Although there is no test that is diagnostic for ankylosing spondylitis, the finding of the HLA B-27 antigen is highly suggestive of the disease in patients with the above clinical findings. This antigen is present in 90% of patients suffering from ankylosing spondylitis. Complete blood cell count may reveal normocytic normochromic anemia. The erythrocyte sedimentation rate is usually elevated, as are the serum IgA levels.

DIFFERENTIAL DIAGNOSIS

Ankylosing spondylitis is a radiographic diagnosis that is supported by a combination of clinical history, physical examination, and laboratory testing. Pain syndromes that may mimic ankylosing spondylitis include low back strain, lumbar bursitis, lumbar fibromyositis, inflammatory arthritis, Reiter's syndrome, the collagen vascular diseases, and disorders of the lumbar spinal cord, roots, plexus, and nerves. Screening laboratory testing consisting of complete blood cell count, erythrocyte sedimentation rate, antinuclear antibody testing, HLA B-27 antigen screening, and automated blood chemistry testing should be performed if the diagnosis of ankylosing spondylitis is in question to help rule out other causes of the patient's pain.

TREATMENT

Ankylosing spondylitis is best treated with a multimodality approach. Physical therapy, including exercises to maintain function, heat modalities, and deep sedative massage, combined with nonsteroidal anti-inflammatory agents and skeletal muscle relaxants represent a reasonable starting point. Sulfasalazine may also be useful in managing the arthritis associated with the disease. The addition of steroid epidural nerve blocks is a reasonable next step. Caudal or lumbar epidural blocks with a local anesthetic and steroid have been shown to be extremely effective in the treatment of pain secondary to ankylosing spondylitis. Underlying sleep disturbance and depression are best treated with a tricyclic antidepressant compound such as nortriptyline, which can be started at a single bedtime dose of 25 mg. Acute uveitis should be managed with corticosteroids and mydriatic agents.

COMPLICATIONS AND PITFALLS

Failure to accurately diagnose ankylosing spondylitis may put the patient at risk for the development of significant functional disability. Myelopathy, which may progress to paraplegia or quadriplegia, is a serious problem if diagnosis is delayed. Electromyography will help sort out plexopathy from radiculopathy and also help identify coexistent entrapment neuropathy such as tarsal tunnel syndrome that confuse the diagnosis.

CLINICAL PEARLS

The diagnosis of ankylosing spondylitis should be considered in any patient complaining of back and/or sacroiliac pain and stiffness that is worse in the morning or after prolonged periods of inactivity. Patients with symptoms of myelopathy should undergo MRI on an urgent basis. Physical therapy combined with nonsteroidal anti-inflammatory agents may help prevent recurrent episodes of pain and help preserve function.

X Pelvic Pain Syndromes

47 *Orchialgia*

THE CLINICAL SYNDROME

Orchialgia, or testicular pain, can be a difficult clinical situation for the patient and clinician alike due to the unique significance the testicle has as part of the male psyche. This fact is crucial if the clinician is to successfully evaluate and treat patients who present with orchialgia.

Acute orchialgia represents a medical emergency and may be the result of trauma, infection or inflammation of the testes or torsion of the testes and spermatic cord.

Chronic orchialgia is defined as testicular pain that is of more than 3 months' duration and significantly interferes with the patient's activities of daily living. Chronic orchialgia can be the result of either pathological processes that are extrascrotal (e.g., ureteral calculi, inguinal hernia, ilioinguinal or genitofemoral nerve entrapment), of diseases of the lumbar spine and roots, or intrascrotal in origin (e.g., chronic epididymides, hydrocele, varicocele). The history of all patients suffering from chronic orchialgia should include specific questioning regarding a past history of sexual abuse.

SIGNS AND SYMPTOMS

Physical examination of patients suffering from acute orchialgia is directed at identifying acute torsion of the testes and spermatic cord, which is a surgical emergency. Patients with acute orchitis secondary to infections including sexually transmitted diseases present with testes that are exquisitely tender to palpation. For patients with chronic orchialgia, the physical findings are often nonspecific with the testicle mildly tender to palpation unless specific pathological processes are present (Fig. 47–1). For example, patients with chronic testicular pain secondary to varicocele will present with a scrotum that feels like a "bag of worms." Patients with chronic epididymitis will present with tenderness that is localized to the epididymis. Testicular malignancy should always be considered in any patient presenting with orchialgia. Physical findings in this setting vary, but testicular enlargement is often an early finding.

As mentioned, extrascrotal pathological processes can also present with the primary symptom of orchialgia. One of the most common causes of orchialgia of extrascrotal origin is ilioinguinal and/or genitofemoral neuralgia. Ilioinguinal neuralgia presents as a sensory deficit in the inner thigh and scrotum in the distribution of the ilioinguinal nerve. Weakness of the anterior abdominal wall musculature may be present. Tinel's sign may be elicited by tapping over the ilioinguinal nerve at the point it pierces the transverse abdominus muscle. The patient suffering from ilioinguinal and/or genitofemoral neuralgia may assume a bent forward novice skier's position to remove pressure on the affected nerve.

TESTING

Ultrasound examination of the scrotal contents is indicated in all patients suffering from orchialgia. Radionucleotide and Doppler studies are indicated if vascular compromise is suspected. Transillumination of the scrotal contents can also help identify varicocele.

Electromyography will help distinguish ilioinguinal nerve entrapment from lumbar plexopathy, lumbar radiculopathy, and diabetic polyneuropathy. Based on the patient's clinical presentation, additional testing including complete blood cell count, uric acid, sedimentation rate, and antinuclear antibody testing may be indicated. Magnetic resonance imaging (MRI) of the lumbar plexus is indicated if tumor or hematoma is suspected.

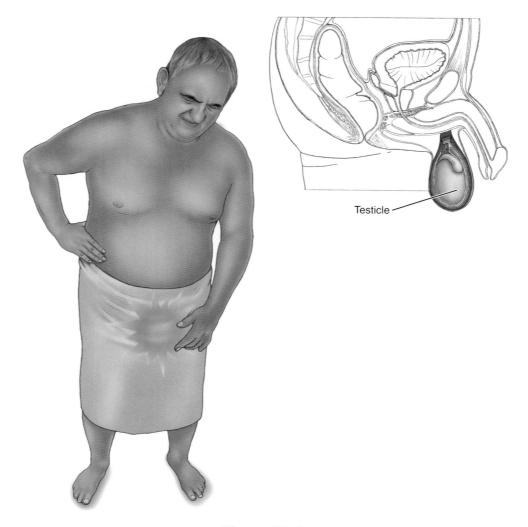

Testicle

Figure 47–1

DIFFERENTIAL DIAGNOSIS

It should be remembered that extrascrotal pathology, including inguinal hernia, ilioinguinal neuralgia, and lesions of the lumbar plexus, nerve roots, and spinal cord, can mimic the pain of orchialgia and must be included in the differential diagnosis. Furthermore, there is significant intrapatient variability in the anatomy of the ilioinguinal and genitofemoral nerves, which can result in significant variation in the patient's clinical presentation. The ilioinguinal nerve is a branch of the L1 nerve root with contribution from T12 in some patients. The nerve follows a curvilinear course that takes it from its origin of the L1 and occasionally T12 somatic nerves to inside the concavity of the ilium. The ilioinguinal nerve continues anteriorly to perforate the transverse abdominis muscle at the level of the anterior superior iliac spine. The nerve may interconnect with the iliohypogastric nerve as it continues to pass along its course medially and inferiorly, where it accompanies the spermatic cord through the inguinal ring and into the inguinal canal. The distribution of the sensory innervation of the ilioinguinal nerves varies from patient to patient as there may be considerable overlap with the iliohypogastric nerve. In general, the ilioinguinal nerve provides sensory innervation to the upper portion of the skin of the inner thigh and the root of the penis and upper scrotum in men.

TREATMENT

Initial treatment of the pain associated with orchialgia should include a combination of the nonsteroidal anti-inflammatory agents or cyclooxygenase-2 (COX-2) inhibitors and physical therapy. The local application of heat and cold may also be beneficial. The use of supportive undergarments or an athletic supporter may also provide symptomatic relief. For patients who do not respond to these treatment modalities, injection of the spermatic cord and/or ilioinguinal and genitofemoral nerves with a local anesthetic and steroid may be a reasonable next step. If the symptoms of orchialgia persist, surgical exploration of the scrotal contents should be considered. Psychological evaluation and interventions should take place concurrently with the above treatment modalities.

COMPLICATIONS AND PITFALLS

The major pitfalls in the care of the patient suffering from orchialgia are fourfold: (1) the misdiagnosis of extrascrotal pathology responsible for the patient's pain; (2) the failure to identify testicular malignancy; (3) the failure to identify vascular compromise or infectious causes of acute orchialgia; and (4) the failure to address the psychological issues surrounding the patient's pain.

CLINICAL PEARLS

The clinician should be aware that the unique relationship of the genitalia to the male psyche presents some unique challenges for the clinician treating patients suffering from orchialgia. The behavioral and psychological issues must be addressed concurrently with the medical issues if success is to be obtained. The possibility for testicular malignancy remains ever present and should be carefully sought out in all patients suffering from orchialgia.

48 *Proctalgia Fugax*

ICD-9 CODE 564.6

THE CLINICAL SYNDROME

Proctalgia fugax is a disease of unknown etiology that is characterized by paroxysms of rectal pain with pain-free periods between attacks. The pain-free periods between attacks can last seconds to minutes. Like cluster headache, spontaneous remissions of the disease occur and may last from weeks to years. Proctalgia fugax is more common in females and occurs with greater frequency in those patients suffering from irritable bowel syndrome.

The pain of proctalgia fugax is sharp or gripping in nature and is severe in intensity. Like other urogenital focal pain syndromes such as vulvadynia and prostadynia, the causes remain obscure. Increased stress will often increase the frequency and intensity of attacks of proctalgia fugax as will sitting for prolonged periods. Patients will often feel an urge to defecate with the onset of the paroxysms of pain (Fig. 48–1). Depression often accompanies the pain of proctalgia fugax but is not thought to be the primary cause. The symptoms of proctalgia fugax can be so severe as to limit the patient's ability to carry out activities of daily living.

SIGNS AND SYMPTOMS

The physical examination of the patient suffering from proctalgia fugax is usually normal. The patient may be depressed or appear anxious. Rectal examination is normal, although deep palpation of the surrounding musculature may trigger paroxysms of pain. Interestingly, the patient suffering from proctalgia fugax will often report that they can abort the attack of pain by placing a finger in the rectum. Rectal suppositories may also interrupt the attacks.

TESTING

As with the physical examination, testing in patients suffering from proctalgia fugax is usually within normal limits. Because of the risk of overlooking rectal malignancy that may be responsible for pain that may be attributed to a benign etiology, by necessity proctalgia fugax must be a diagnosis of exclusion. Rectal examination is mandatory in all patients thought to be suffering from proctalgia fugax. Sigmoidoscopy or colonoscopy is also strongly recommended in such patients. Testing of the stool of occult blood is also indicated. Screening laboratory studies consisting of a complete blood cell count, automated chemistries, and erythrocyte sedimentation rate should also be performed. Magnetic resonance imaging (MRI) or computed tomography (CT) scanning of the pelvis should also be considered if the diagnosis is in doubt. If psychological problems are suspected or if there is a history of sexual abuse, psychiatric evaluation is indicated concurrently with laboratory and radiographic testing.

DIFFERENTIAL DIAGNOSIS

As mentioned, because of the risk of overlooking serious pathology of the anus and rectum, proctalgia fugax must be a diagnosis of exclusion. First and foremost, the clinician must rule out rectal malignancy to avoid disaster. Proctitis can mimic the pain of proctalgia fugax and can be diagnosed on sigmoidoscopy or colonoscopy. Hemorrhoids will usually present with bleeding associated with pain and can be distinguished from proctalgia fugax on physical examination. Prostadynia may sometimes be confused with proctalgia fugax, but the pain is more constant and duller and aching in character.

176

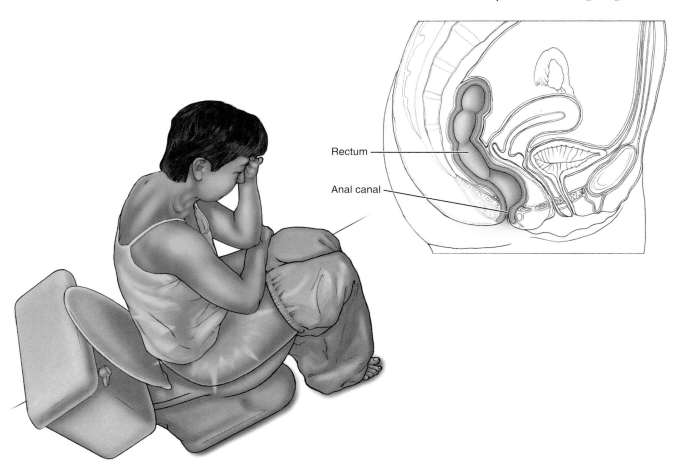

Rectum

Anal canal

Figure 48–1

TREATMENT

Initial treatment of proctalgia fugax should include a combination of simple analgesics and the non-steroidal anti-inflammatory agents or the cyclooxygenase-2 (COX-2) inhibitors. If these medications do not adequately control the patient's symptomatology, a tricyclic antidepressant or gabapentin should be added.

Traditionally, the tricyclic antidepressants have been a mainstay in the palliation of pain secondary to proctalgia fugax. Controlled studies have demonstrated the efficacy of amitriptyline for this indication. Other tricyclic antidepressants including nortriptyline and desipramine have also shown to be clinically useful. Unfortunately, this class of drugs is associated with significant anticholinergic side effects, including dry mouth, constipation, sedation, and urinary retention. These drugs should be used with caution in those suffering from glaucoma, cardiac arrhythmia, and prostatism. To minimize side effects and encourage compliance, the primary care physician should start amitriptyline or nortriptyline at a 10-mg dose at bedtime. The dose can be then titrated upward to 25 mg at bedtime as side effects allow. Upward titration of dosage in 25-mg increments can be carried out each week as side effects allow. Even at lower doses, patients will generally report a rapid improvement in sleep disturbance and will begin to experience some pain relief in 10 to 14 days. If the patient does not experience any improvement in pain as the dose is being titrated upward, the addition of gabapentin alone or in combination with nerve blocks of the intercostal nerves with local anesthetics and/or steroid is recommended. The selective serotonin reuptake inhibitors such as fluoxetine have also be used to treat the pain of diabetic neuropathy, and although better tolerated than the tricyclic antidepressants, they appear to be less efficacious.

If the antidepressant compounds are ineffective or contraindicated, gabapentin represents a reasonable alternative. Gabapentin should be started with a 300-mg dose of gabapentin at bedtime for 2 nights. The patient should be cautioned about potential side effects, including dizziness, sedation, confusion, and rash. The drug is then increased in 300-mg incre-ments, given in equally divided doses over 2 days, as side effects allow until pain relief is obtained or a total dose of 2400 mg daily is reached. At this point, if the patient has experienced partial relief of pain, blood values are measured and the drug is carefully titrated upward using 100-mg tablets. Rarely will more than 3600 mg daily be required.

The local application of heat and cold may also be beneficial to provide symptomatic relief of the pain of proctalgia fugax. The use of bland rectal suppositories may also help provide symptomatic relief. For patients who do not respond to these treatment modalities, injection of the peroneal nerves or caudal epidural nerve block using a local anesthetic and steroid may be a reasonable next step. The clinician should be aware that there are anecdotal reports that the calcium channel blockers, topical nitroglycerin, and inhalation of albuterol will provide symptomatic relief of the pain of proctalgia fugax.

COMPLICATIONS AND PITFALLS

The major problem in the care of patients thought to suffer from proctalgia fugax is the failure to identify potentially serious pathology of the anus or rectum due to primary tumor or invasion of these structures by pelvic tumor. Although uncommon, occult rectal infection remains a possibility, especially in the immunocompromised patient with cancer. Early detection of infection is crucial to avoid potentially life-threatening sequelae.

CLINICAL PEARLS

Proctalgia fugax is a distressing disease for the patient. The paroxysms of pain may appear without warning and make the patient afraid to leave the house. The main focus of the clinician caring for the patient suffering from proctalgia fugax is to ensure that occult malignancy has not been overlooked. Given the psychological implications of pain involving the genitals and rectum, the clinician should not overlook the possibility of psychological abnormality in patients with pain in the rectum.

49 *Prostadynia*

ICD-9 CODE 608.9

THE CLINICAL SYNDROME

Prostadynia is an uncommon cause of perineal pain in the male. Also known as *chronic nonbacterial prostatitis/chronic pelvic pain syndrome (CNP/CPPS)*, prostadynia probably is not a single clinical entity but rather the conglomeration of a variety of disorders that can cause pain in this anatomic region. Included in these disorders are chronic infections of the prostate, chronic inflammation of the prostate without demonstrable infection, bladder outflow abnormalities, pelvic floor muscle disorders, reflex sympathetic dystrophy, and psychogenic causes. All have in common the ability to cause chronic, ill-defined perineal pain, which is the hallmark of prostadynia.

The pain of prostadynia is characterized by dull, aching, or burning pain of the perineum and underlying structures (Fig. 49–1). The intensity of pain is mild to moderate and may worsen with urination or sexual activity. The pain may be referred to the penis, testicles, scrotum, or inner thigh. Irritative urinary outflow symptoms and sexual dysfunction often coexist with the pain of prostadynia. The history of all patients suffering from chronic prostadynia should include specific questioning regarding a past history of sexual abuse.

SIGNS AND SYMPTOMS

Physical examination of patients suffering from acute prostadynia is directed at identifying acute bacterial infection of the prostate and/or urinary tract. Patients with acute orchitis secondary to infections including sexually transmitted diseases will present with a prostate that is exquisitely tender to palpation.

For patients with chronic prostadynia, the physical findings are often nonspecific with the prostate mildly tender to palpation unless specific pathological processes are present. Allodynia of the perineum is also often present. Prostate malignancy should always be considered in any patient presenting with prostadynia. Physical findings in this setting vary, but prostate enlargement is often an early finding.

Extraprostate pathological processes can also occur with the primary symptom of prostadynia. One of the most common causes of prostadynia of extraprostate origin is malignancy involving the pelvic contents other than the prostate. Tumor involving the lumbar plexus, cauda equina, and/or hypogastric plexus can rarely present as pain localized to the prostate and perineum. Postradiation neuropathy can occur after radiation therapy for the treatment of malignancy of the prostate and rectum and can mimic the pain of prostadynia.

TESTING

Digital examination of the prostate is the cornerstone of the diagnosis of patients suffering from prostadynia. Careful examination for tenderness, nodules, and/or tumor is crucial to avoid overlooking prostatic malignancy. Ultrasound examination of the prostate is indicated in all patients suffering from prostadynia. If there is any question of occult malignancy of the prostate or pelvic contents, magnetic resonance imaging (MRI) or computed tomography (CT) scanning of the pelvis is mandatory, as is laboratory determination of the prostatic specific antigen level. It should be noted that acute infection of the prostate can elevate the prostatic specific antigen level. Urinalysis to rule out urinary tract infection is also indicated in all patients suffering from prostadynia. The role of laboratory examination of postprostatic massage prostatic fluid in the evaluation of prostadynia remains unclear, although there are anecdotal reports of the consistent finding of an

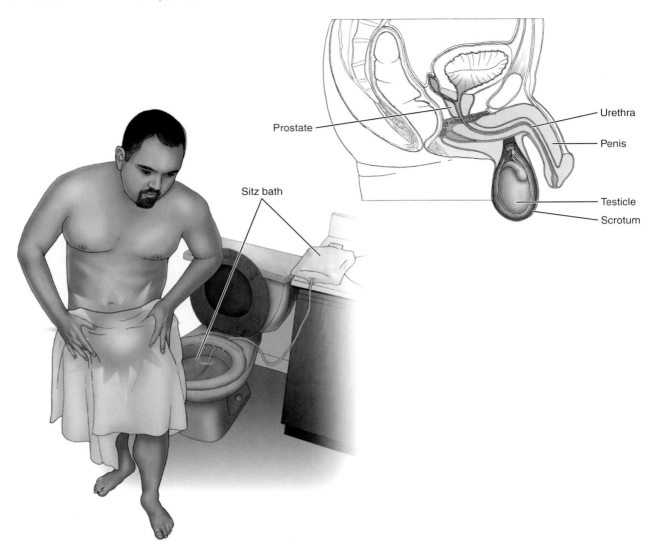

Sitz bath

Prostate

Urethra

Penis

Testicle

Scrotum

Figure 49–1

elevated uric acid level in the prostatic fluid of patients suffering from prostadynia.

Electromyography will help distinguish radiation neuropathy from lumbar plexopathy or lumbar radiculopathy. Based on the patient's clinical presentation, additional testing including complete blood cell count, uric acid, sedimentation rate, and antinuclear antibody testing may be indicated. MRI of the lumbar plexus is indicated if tumor or hematoma is suspected.

DIFFERENTIAL DIAGNOSIS

It should be remembered that extraprostate pathology, including reflex sympathetic dystrophy and lesions of the lumbar plexus, nerve roots, and spinal cord, can mimic the pain of prostadynia and must be included in the differential diagnosis. As mentioned, because of the disastrous results of missing a diagnosis of prostatic malignancy when evaluating and treating patients thought to be suffering from prostadynia, it is mandatory that malignancy be high on the list of differential diagnostic possibilities (Fig. 49–2).

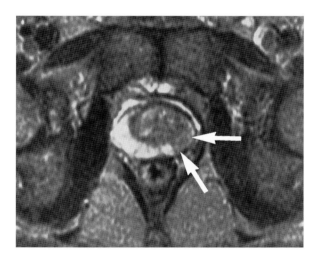

Figure 49–2. Prostate cancer (*arrows*) infiltrating and displacing the normal high–signal intensity peripheral zone. The fibrous prostate capsule is intact, separating the cancer from the high–signal intensity lateral periprostatic venous plexus. (From Stark DD, Bradley WG Jr: Magnetic Resonance Imaging, 3rd ed. St Louis, Mosby, 1999, p 626.)

TREATMENT

Initial treatment of the pain associated with prostadynia should include a combination of the nonsteroidal anti-inflammatory agents or cyclooxygenase-2 (COX-2) inhibitors. The local application of heat and cold via sitz baths may also be beneficial. An arbitrary treatment course of antibiotics such as doxycycline 100 mg twice a day for 2 weeks may also be worth a try even though urine cultures are negative. Anecdotal reports of decreased pain after treatment with allopurinol make this drug a consideration for patients who continue to have pain.

For patients who do not respond to these treatment modalities, caudal epidural block nerves with a local anesthetic and steroid may be a reasonable next step. Psychological evaluation and interventions should take place concurrently with the above treatment modalities given the high incidence of coexistent psychological issues associated with all pelvic pain syndromes.

COMPLICATIONS AND PITFALLS

The major pitfalls in the care of the patient suffering from prostadynia are threefold: (1) the misdiagnosis of extraprostate pathology responsible for the patient's pain; (2) the failure to identify prostate malignancy; and (3) the failure to address the psychological issues surrounding the patient's pain.

CLINICAL PEARLS

The clinician should be aware that the unique relationship of the genitalia to the male psyche presents some unique challenges for the clinician treating patients suffering from prostadynia. The behavioral and psychological issues must be addressed concurrently with the medical issues if success is to be obtained. The possibility for prostate malignancy remains ever present and should be carefully sought out in all patients suffering from prostadynia.

50 *Vulvadynia*

THE CLINICAL SYNDROME

Vulvadynia is an uncommon cause of pelvic pain encountered in clinical practice. Vulvadynia probably is not a single clinical entity but rather the conglomeration of a variety of disorders that can cause pain in this anatomical region. Included in these disorders are chronic infections of the female urogenital tract; chronic inflammation of the skin and mucosa of the vulva without demonstrable bacterial, viral, or fungal infection; and bladder abnormalities including interstitial cystitis, pelvic floor muscle disorders, reflex sympathetic dystrophy, and psychogenic causes. All have in common the ability to cause chronic, ill-defined pain of the vulva that is the hallmark of vulvadynia.

The pain of vulvadynia is characterized by dull, stinging, aching, or burning pain of the vulva. The intensity of pain is mild to moderate and may worsen with bathing, urination, or sexual activity. The pain may be referred to the perineum, rectum, or inner thigh. Irritative urinary outflow symptoms and sexual dysfunction often coexist with the pain of vulvadynia, with vulvadynia being one of the leading causes of dyspareunia (Fig. 50–1). The history of all patients suffering from chronic vulvadynia should include specific questioning regarding a past history of sexual abuse, sexually transmitted diseases, and psychological abnormalities related to sexuality.

SIGNS AND SYMPTOMS

Physical examination of patients suffering from acute vulvadynia is directed at identifying acute infections of the vulva and/or urinary tract that may be readily treatable. Patients with acute infections, including yeast infections and sexually transmitted diseases, will present with a vulva that is irritated, inflamed, raw to the touch, and tender to palpation. For patients with chronic vulvadynia, the physical findings are often nonspecific, with the vulva mildly tender to palpation and an otherwise normal pelvic examination. Changes of the skin and mucous membranes of the vulva due to herpes, chronic itching, irritation, or douching may also be present. In a small number of patients suffering from vulvadynia, spasm of the muscles of the pelvic floor may be demonstrated on pelvic examination. Allodynia of the vulva and perineum may be present, especially if there is a history of prior trauma, such as surgery, radiation therapy, straddle injuries, etc. Vulva malignancy should always be considered in any patient presenting with vulvadynia.

Extravulva pathological processes can also present with the primary symptom of vulvadynia. One of the most common causes of vulvadynia of extravulva origin is malignancy involving the pelvic contents other than the vulva. Tumor involving the lumbar plexus, cauda equina, and/or hypogastric plexus can rarely present as pain localized to the vulva and perineum. Postradiation neuropathy can occur after radiation therapy for the treatment of malignancy of the vulva and rectum and can mimic the pain of vulvadynia. Ilioinguinal or genitofemoral entrapment neuropathy can also present clinically as vulvadynia.

TESTING

Pelvic examination is the cornerstone of the diagnosis of patients suffering from vulvadynia. Careful examination for infection, cutaneous or mucosal abnormalities, tenderness, muscle spasm, and/or tumor is crucial to avoid overlooking vulvar malignancy. Ultrasound examination of the pelvis is indicated in all patients suffering from vulvadynia. If there is any question of occult malignancy of the vulva or pelvic contents, magnetic resonance

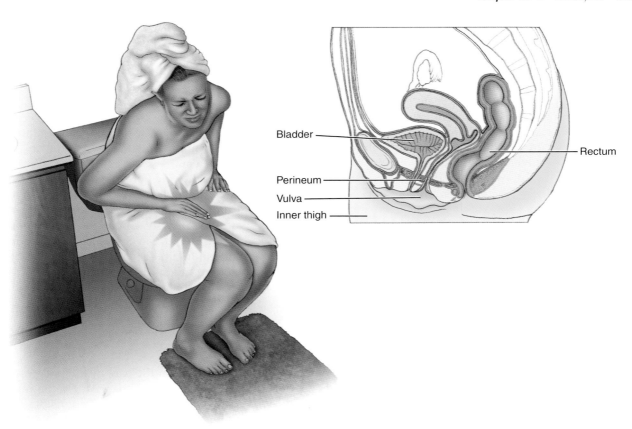

Bladder

Perineum

Vulva

Inner thigh

Rectum

Figure 50–1

imaging (MRI) or computed tomography (CT) scanning of the pelvis is mandatory to rule out malignancy or disease of the pelvic organs, such as endometriosis, that may be responsible for the patient's pain symptomatology. Urinalysis to rule out urinary tract infection is also indicated in all patients suffering from vulvadynia. Culture for sexually transmitted diseases including herpes is also indicated in the evaluation of all patients thought to be suffering from vulvadynia.

Electromyography will help distinguish entrapment neuropathy of the genitofemoral or ilioinguinal nerves from lumbar plexopathy or lumbar radiculopathy. Based on the patient's clinical presentation, additional testing including complete blood cell count, sedimentation rate, and antinuclear antibody testing may be indicated. MRI of the lumbar plexus is indicated if tumor or hematoma is suspected.

DIFFERENTIAL DIAGNOSIS

It should be remembered that extravulvar pathology, including reflex sympathetic dystrophy and lesions of the lumbar plexus, nerve roots, and spinal cord, can mimic the pain of vulvadynia and must be included in the differential diagnosis. As mentioned, because of the disastrous results of missing a diagnosis of pelvic or vulvar malignancy when evaluating and treating patients thought to be suffering from vulvadynia, it is mandatory that malignancy be high on the list of differential diagnostic possibilities.

TREATMENT

Initial treatment of the pain associated with vulvadynia should include a combination of the nonsteroidal anti-inflammatory agents or cyclooxygenase-2 (COX-2) inhibitors. The local application of heat and cold via sitz baths may also be beneficial. An arbitrary treatment course of antibiotics such as doxycycline 100 mg twice a day for 2 weeks may also be worth a try even though urine cultures are negative. A course of treatment for vaginal yeast infection concurrently with the antibiotics should also be considered. Anecdotal reports of decreased pain after treatment with adjuvant analgesics such as the tricyclic antidepressants, such as nortriptyline at 25 mg at bedtime and titrating upward as side effects allow or gabapentin, make these drugs a consideration for patients who continue to have pain in the absence of demonstrable treatable disease.

For patients who do not respond to these treatment modalities, caudal epidural block nerves with a local anesthetic and steroid may be a reasonable next step. If the symptoms of vulvadynia persist, laparoscopy should be considered. Psychological evaluation and interventions should take place concurrently with the above treatment modalities given the high incidence of coexistent psychological issues associated with all pelvic pain syndromes.

COMPLICATIONS AND PITFALLS

The major pitfalls in the care of the patient suffering from vulvadynia are threefold: (1) the misdiagnosis of extravulvar pathology responsible for the patient's pain; (2) the failure to identify vulva and/or pelvic malignancy; and (3) the failure to address the psychological issues surrounding the patient's pain.

CLINICAL PEARLS

The clinician should be aware that the unique relationship of the genitalia to the female psyche presents some unique challenges for the clinician treating patients suffering from vulvadynia. The behavioral and psychological issues must be addressed concurrently with the medical issues if success is to be obtained. The possibility for vulva and/or pelvic malignancy remains ever present and should be carefully sought out in all patients suffering from vulvadynia.

51 *Gluteal Bursitis*

THE CLINICAL SYNDROME

Gluteal bursitis is an uncommon cause of buttock pain that is frequently misdiagnosed as primary hip pathology. The patient suffering from gluteal bursitis will frequently complain of pain at the upper outer quadrant of the buttock and with resisted abduction and extension of the lower extremity. The pain is localized to the area over the upper outer quadrant of the buttock, with referred pain noted into the sciatic notch. Often, the patient will be unable to sleep on the affected hip and may complain of a sharp, catching sensation when extending and abducting the hip, especially on first awakening.

The gluteal bursae lay between the gluteal maximus, medius, and minimus muscles as well as between these muscles and the underlying bone. These bursae may exist as a single bursal sac or in some patients may exist as a multisegmented series of sacs that may be loculated in nature. The gluteal bursae are vulnerable to injury from both acute trauma and repeated microtrauma. The action of the gluteus maximus muscle includes the flexion of trunk on thigh when maintaining a sitting position when riding a horse (Fig. 51–1). This action can irritate the gluteal bursae and result in pain and inflammation. Acute injuries frequently take the form of direct trauma to the bursa from falls directly onto the buttocks or repeated intramuscular injections as well as from overuse such as running for long distances, especially on soft or uneven surfaces. If the inflammation of the gluteal bursae becomes chronic, calcification of the bursae may occur.

SIGNS AND SYMPTOMS

Physical examination of patients suffering from gluteal bursitis may reveal point tenderness in the upper outer quadrant of the buttocks. Passive flexion and adduction as well as active resisted extension and abduction of the affected lower extremity will reproduce the pain. Sudden release of resistance during this maneuver will markedly increase the pain.

Examination of the hip will be within normal limits, as will examination of the sacroiliac joint. Careful neurological examination of the affected lower extremity should reveal no neurological deficits. If neurological deficits are present, evaluation for plexopathy, radiculopathy, or entrapment neuropathy should be undertaken. It should be remembered that these neurological symptoms can coexist with gluteal bursitis, confusing the clinical diagnosis.

TESTING

Plain radiographs of the hip may reveal calcification of the bursa and associated structures consistent with chronic inflammation. Magnetic resonance imaging (MRI) is indicated if occult mass or tumor of the hip is suspected. Electromyography should be performed if neurological findings are present to rule out plexopathy, radiculopathy, and/or nerve entrapment syndromes of the lower extremity. Based on the patient's clinical presentation, additional testing including complete blood cell count, HLA B-27 testing, automated serum chemistries including uric acid, sedimentation rate, and antinuclear antibody testing may be indicated. The injection technique described here serves as both a diagnostic and therapeutic maneuver for patients suffering from gluteal bursitis.

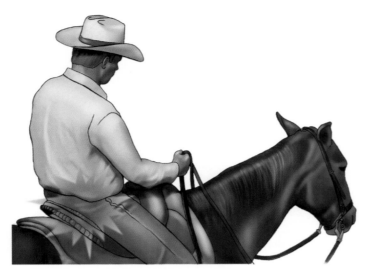

Figure 51-1

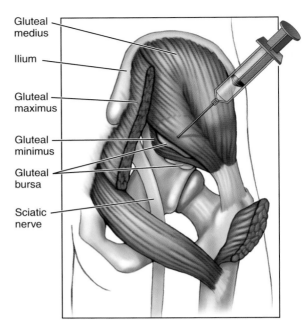

Figure 51-2

TREATMENT

Initial treatment of the pain and functional disability associated with gluteal bursitis should include a combination of the nonsteroidal anti-inflammatory agents or cyclooxygenase-2 (COX-2) inhibitors and physical therapy. The local application of heat and cold may also be beneficial. The repetitive movements that incite the syndrome should be avoided. For patients who do not respond to these treatment modalities, injection of gluteal bursa with a local anesthetic and steroid may be a reasonable next step.

To inject the gluteal bursae, the patient is placed in the lateral position with the affected side up and the affected leg flexed at the knee. Proper preparation with antiseptic solution of the skin overlying the upper outer quadrant of the buttocks is then carried out. A syringe containing 4.0 mL of 0.25% preservative-free bupivacaine and 40 mg of methylprednisolone is attached to a 25-gauge 1½-inch needle. The point of maximal tenderness within the upper outer quadrant of the buttocks is then identified with a sterilely gloved finger. Before needle placement, the patient should be advised to say "There!!!" immediately if they feel a paresthesia into the lower extremity, indicating that the needle has impinged on the sciatic nerve. Should a paresthesia occur, the needle should be immediately withdrawn and repositioned more medially. The needle is then carefully advanced perpendicular to the skin at the previously identified point until it impinges on the wing of the ilium (Fig. 51–2). Care must be taken to keep the needle medial and not to advance it laterally or it could impinge on the sciatic nerve. After careful aspiration and if no paresthesia is present, the contents of the syringe are then gently injected into the bursa. There should be minimal resistance to injection.

DIFFERENTIAL DIAGNOSIS

Gluteal bursitis is often misdiagnosed as sciatica or attributed to primary hip pathology. Radiographs of the hip and electromyography will help distinguish gluteal bursitis from radiculopathy of pain emanating from the hip. Most patients suffering from a lumbar radiculopathy will have back pain associated with reflex, motor, and sensory changes, whereas patients with gluteal bursitis will have only secondary back pain and no neurological changes. Piriformis syndrome may sometimes be confused with gluteal bursitis but can distinguished by the presence of motor and sensory changes involving the sciatic nerve. These motor and sensory changes will be limited to the distribution of the sciatic nerve below the sciatic notch. It should be remembered that lumbar radiculopathy and sciatic nerve entrapment may coexist as the "double crush" syndrome. The pain of gluteal bursitis may cause alteration of gait, which may result in secondary back and radicular symptomatology that may coexist with this entrapment neuropathy.

SIDE EFFECTS AND PITFALLS

The proximity to the sciatic nerve makes it imperative that this procedure be carried out only by those well versed in the regional anatomy and experienced in performing injection techniques. Many patients will also complain of a transient increase in pain after injection of the bursae.

CLINICAL PEARLS

This injection technique is extremely effective in the treatment of gluteal bursitis. This technique is a safe procedure if careful attention is paid to the clinically relevant anatomy in the areas to be injected. Care must be taken to use sterile techniques to avoid infection, as well as the use of universal precautions to avoid risk to the operator. Most side effects of this injection technique are related to needle-induced trauma to the injection site and underlying tissues. The incidence of ecchymosis and hematoma formation can be decreased if pressure is placed on the injection site immediately after injection. The avoidance of overly long needles will help decrease the incidence of trauma to underlying structures. Special care must be taken to avoid trauma to the sciatic nerve.

The use of physical modalities, including local heat as well as gentle stretching exercises, should be introduced several days after the patient undergoes this injection technique. Vigorous exercises should be avoided because they will exacerbate the patient's symptomatology. Simple analgesics, nonsteroidal anti-inflammatory agents, and antimyotonic agents such as tizanidine may be used concurrently with this injection technique.

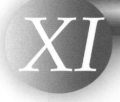

XI

Hip and Lower Extremity Pain Syndromes

52 *Psoas Bursitis*

ICD-9 CODE 727.3

THE CLINICAL SYNDROME

Psoas bursitis is an uncommon cause of hip and groin pain that is frequently misdiagnosed in clinical practice. The patient suffering from psoas bursitis will frequently complain of pain in the groin. The pain is localized to the area just below the crease of the groin anteriorly with referred pain noted into the hip joint. Often, the patient will be unable to sleep on the affected hip and may complain of a sharp, catching sensation with range of motion of the hip.

The psoas muscle flexes the thigh on the trunk or, if the thigh is fixed, flexes the trunk on the thigh as when moving from a supine to sitting position. This action can irritate the psoas bursa as can repeated trauma from repetitive activity including running up stairs or overuse of exercise equipment for lower extremity strengthening (Fig. 52–1). The psoas muscle is innervated by the lumbar plexus. The psoas bursa lies medially in the femoral triangle between the psoas tendon and the anterior aspect of the neck of the femur. This bursa may exist as a single bursal sac or in some patients may exist as a multiseg-mented series of sacs that may be loculated in nature. The psoas bursa is vulnerable to injury from both acute trauma and repeated microtrauma. Acute injuries frequently take the form of direct trauma to the bursa from seat belt injuries as well as from overuse injuries requiring repeated hip flexion such as javelin throwing and ballet. If the inflammation of the psoas bursa becomes chronic, calcification of the bursa may occur.

SIGNS AND SYMPTOMS

Physical examination may reveal point tenderness in the upper thigh just below the crease of the groin in patients suffering from psoas bursitis. Passive flexion, adduction, and abduction as well as active resisted flexion and adduction of the affected lower extremity will reproduce the pain. Sudden release of resistance during this maneuver will markedly increase the pain. Examination of the hip will be within normal limits unless there is coexistent internal derangement of the hip.

TESTING

Plain radiographs of the hip may reveal calcification of the bursa and associated structures consistent with chronic inflammation. Magnetic resonance imaging (MRI) is indicated if occult mass or tumor of the hip or groin is suspected. Complete blood cell count, automated chemistry profile including uric acid, sedimentation rate, and antinuclear antibody testing is indicated if collagen vascular disease is suspected. Injection of the psoas bursae with a local anesthetic and steroid serves as both a diagnostic and therapeutic maneuver.

DIFFERENTIAL DIAGNOSIS

Psoas bursitis is often misdiagnosed as an inguinal hernia or attributed to primary hip pathology. Radiographs of the hip and electromyography will help distinguish psoas bursitis from radiculopathy of pain emanating from the hip. Most patients suffering from a lumbar radiculopathy will have back pain associated with reflex, motor, and sensory changes, whereas patients with psoas bursitis will have only secondary back pain due to altered gait and no neurological changes. Femoral diabetic neuropathy may sometimes be confused with psoas bursitis but can be distinguished by the presence of motor and sensory changes involving the femoral nerve. These motor and sensory changes will be limited to the distribution of the femoral nerve below the inguinal

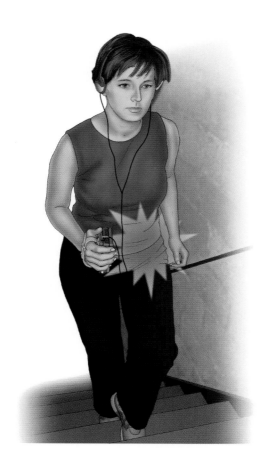

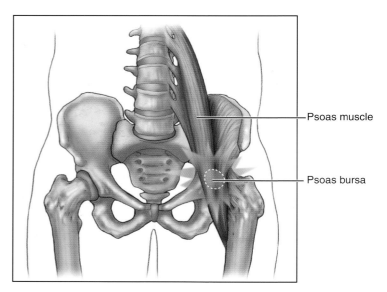

Psoas muscle

Psoas bursa

Figure 52–1

ligament. Ilioinguinal and genitofemoral neuropathy can also be confused with psoas bursitis. It should be remembered that lumbar radiculopathy and these nerve entrapments may coexist as the "double crush" syndrome. The pain of psoas bursitis may also cause alteration of gait, which may result in secondary back and radicular symptomatology that may coexist with this entrapment neuropathy.

TREATMENT

Initial treatment of the pain and functional disability associated with psoas bursitis should include a combination of the nonsteroidal anti-inflammatory agents or cyclooxygenase-2 (COX-2) inhibitors and physical therapy. The local application of heat and cold may also be beneficial. The repetitive movements that incite the syndrome should be avoided. For patients who do not respond to these treatment modalities, injection of psoas bursa with a local anesthetic and steroid may be a reasonable next step.

SIDE EFFECTS AND PITFALLS

The proximity to the femoral nerve of the psoas bursa makes it imperative that this procedure be carried out only by those well versed in the regional anatomy and experienced in performing injection techniques. Many patients will also complain of a transient increase in pain after injection of the bursae.

CLINICAL PEARLS

It is important to rule out other causes of groin pain including inguinal hernia and entrapment neuropathies of the ilioinguinal, genitofemoral, and femoral nerves. Injection of the psoas bursae is extremely effective in the treatment of psoas bursitis. Special care must be taken to avoid trauma to the femoral nerve.

The use of physical modalities, including local heat as well as gentle stretching exercises, should be introduced several days after the patient undergoes this injection technique. Vigorous exercises should be avoided because they will exacerbate the patient's symptomatology. Simple analgesics, nonsteroidal anti-inflammatory agents, and antimyotonic agents such as tizanidine may be used concurrently with injection of the bursae.

53 *Femoral Neuropathy*

ICD-9 CODE 355.8

THE CLINICAL SYNDROME

Femoral neuropathy is an uncommon cause of anterior thigh and medial calf pain that has many etiologies. Femoral neuropathy may be due to compression by tumor, retroperitoneal hemorrhage, or abscess. Stretch injuries to the femoral nerve as it passes under the inguinal ligament from extreme extension or flexion at the hip may also produce the symptoms of femoral neuropathy. Direct trauma to the nerve from surgery or during cardiac catheterization can also produce this clinical syndrome, as can diabetes, which can produce vascular lesions of the nerve itself.

The patient with femoral neuropathy presents with pain that radiates into the anterior thigh and midcalf and is associated with weakness of the quadriceps muscle. This weakness can result in significant functional deficit with the patient being unable to fully extend the knee, which can allow the knee to buckle, resulting in inexplicable falls. The patient suffering from femoral neuropathy may also experience weakness of the hip flexors, making walking up stairs quite difficult.

SIGNS AND SYMPTOMS

The patient with femoral neuropathy will present with pain that radiates into the anterior thigh and medial calf (Fig. 53–1). This pain may be paresthetic or burning in character. The intensity is moderate to severe. Weakness of the quadriceps muscle can be quite marked, and over time atrophy of the quadriceps may occur, especially in diabetic patients. Patients with femoral neuropathy may complain of a sunburned feeling over the anterior thigh. The

patient may also complain that their knee feels like it is giving away.

TESTING

Electromyography can help identify the exact source of neurological dysfunction and help clarify the differential diagnosis and thus should be the starting point of the evaluation of all patients suspected of having femoral neuropathy. Plain radiographs of the spine, hip, and pelvis are indicated in all patients who present with femoral neuropathy to rule out occult bony pathology. Based on the patient's clinical presentation, additional testing including complete blood cell count, uric acid, sedimentation rate, and antinuclear antibody testing may be indicated. Magnetic resonance imaging (MRI) of the spine and pelvis is indicated if tumor or hematoma is suspected. Injection of the femoral nerve at the femoral triangle serves as both a diagnostic and therapeutic maneuver.

DIFFERENTIAL DIAGNOSIS

It is difficult to separate femoral neuropathy from a L4 radiculopathy on purely clinical grounds. There may be subtle differences in that the L4 radiculopathy may present with sensory changes into the foot and weakness of the dorsiflexors of the foot. It should be remembered that intrapelvic or retroperitoneal tumor or hematoma may compress the lumbar plexus and mimic the clinical presentation of femoral neuropathy.

TREATMENT

Mild cases of femoral neuropathy will usually respond to conservative therapy, and surgery should be reserved for more severe cases. Initial treatment of femoral neuropathy should consist of treatment with

194

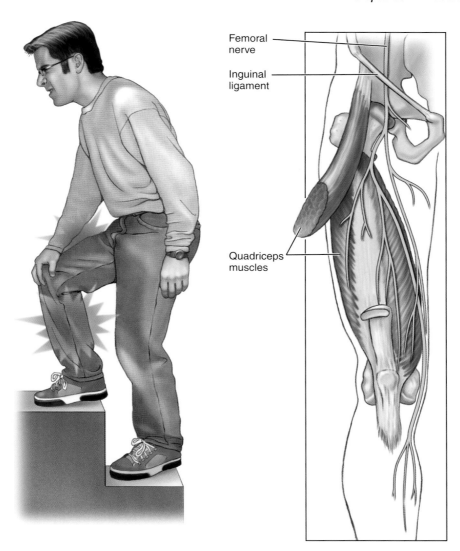

Figure 53–1

simple analgesics, nonsteroidal anti-inflammatory agents, or cyclooxygenase-2 (COX-2) inhibitors and avoidance of repetitive activities that exacerbate the patient's symptomatology. If diabetes is thought to be the etiology of the patient's femoral neuropathy, tight control of blood sugars is mandatory. Avoidance of repetitive activities thought to be responsible for the exacerbation of femoral neuropathy (e.g., repetitive hip extension and flexion, etc.) will also help ameliorate the patient's symptoms. If the patient fails to respond to these conservative measures, a next reasonable step is injection of the femoral nerve with a local anesthetic and steroid.

SIDE EFFECTS AND PITFALLS

It is imperative that the clinician rules out causes of femoral neuropathy that, if undiagnosed, could harm the patient, such as uncontrolled diabetes and retroperitoneal or pelvic tumor. The main side effect of femoral nerve block is postblock ecchymosis and hematoma. The potential for needle-induced trauma to the femoral nerve remains a possibility. By advancing the needle slowly and then withdrawing the needle slightly away from the nerve, needle-induced trauma to the femoral nerve can be avoided.

CLINICAL PEARLS

Femoral neuropathy should always be differentiated from lumbar plexopathy and radiculopathy of the nerve roots that may at times mimic femoral nerve compression. Furthermore, it should be remembered that lumbar radiculopathy and femoral nerve entrapment may coexist in the "double crush" syndrome. The double crush syndrome is seen most commonly with median nerve entrapment at the wrist.

Injection of the femoral nerve is a simple and safe technique in the evaluation and treatment of the above-mentioned painful conditions. Careful neurological examination to identify preexisting neurological deficits that may later be attributed to the nerve block should be performed on all patients before beginning femoral nerve block, especially in those patients with clinical symptoms of diabetes or clinically significant femoral neuropathy.

54 Obturator Neuralgia

ICD-9 CODE 355.8

THE CLINICAL SYNDROME

Obturator neuralgia is an uncommon cause of medial thigh pain that does not extend below the knee and occurs most often after trauma. Pelvic fractures, gunshot wounds, and occasionally childbirth have been implicated in the evolution of obturator neuralgia. With the increased number of total hip arthroplasties being performed, trauma to the branches of the obturator nerve may occur, producing pain and numbness over the medial thigh. Obturator neuralgia may also be due to compression of the nerve by tumor, hemorrhage, bone cement from total hip arthroplasties, or abscess. Stretch injuries to the obturator nerve can also cause the symptoms of obturator neuralgia. Diabetes can also affect the obturator nerve, but this is usually in conjunction with neuropathy of the other nerves of the lower extremity, especially the femoral nerve.

SIGNS AND SYMPTOMS

The patient with obturator neuralgia will present with pain that radiates into the medial thigh and, except in rare patients, does not extend below the knee (Fig. 54–1). This pain may be paresthetic or burning in character. The intensity is moderate to severe. There is no significant motor deficit associated with obturator neuralgia unless the spinal nerve roots, plexus, or other peripheral nerves are involved. Patients with obturator neuralgia may complain of a sunburned feeling over the distribution of the obturator nerve.

TESTING

Electromyography can help identify the exact source of neurological dysfunction and help clarify the differential diagnosis and thus should be the starting point of the evaluation of all patients suspected of having obturator neuralgia. Plain radiographs of the spine, hip, pelvis, and proximal femur are indicated in all patients who present with obturator neuralgia to rule out occult bony pathology. Based on the patient's clinical presentation, additional testing including complete blood cell count, uric acid, sedimentation rate, and antinuclear antibody testing may be indicated. Magnetic resonance imaging (MRI) of the spine, pelvis, and proximal lower extremity is indicated if tumor or hematoma is suspected. Injection of the obturator nerve with a local anesthetic and steroid serves as both a diagnostic and therapeutic maneuver.

DIFFERENTIAL DIAGNOSIS

It is sometimes difficult to separate obturator neuralgia from a lumbar plexopathy or radiculopathy on purely clinical grounds, and electromyography is strongly recommended. Electromyography and nerve conduction testing will also help rule out the presence of peripheral neuropathy. It should be remembered that intrapelvic or retroperitoneal tumor or hematoma may compress the lumbar plexus and mimic the clinical presentation of obturator neuralgia.

TREATMENT

Mild cases of obturator neuralgia will usually respond to conservative therapy, and surgery should be reserved for more severe cases. Initial treatment of obturator neuralgia should consist of treatment with simple analgesics, nonsteroidal anti-inflammatory agents, or cyclooxygenase-2 (COX-2) inhibitors and avoidance of repetitive activities that exacerbate the patient's symptomatology. If diabetes is thought to be the etiology of the patient's obturator neuralgia, tight

197

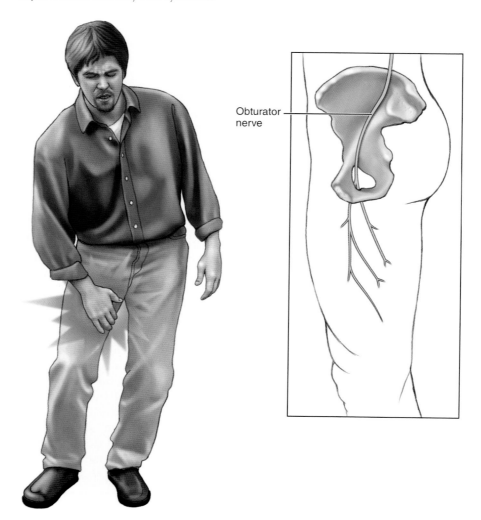

Figure 54–1

control of blood sugar levels is mandatory. Avoidance of repetitive activities thought to be responsible for the exacerbation of obturator neuralgia will also help ameliorate the patient's symptoms. The use of gabapentin or a tricyclic antidepressant such as nortriptyline as an adjuvant analgesic may also help ameliorate the symptoms of obturator neuralgia. If the patient fails to respond to these conservative measures, a next reasonable step is injection of the obturator nerve with a local anesthetic and steroid.

SIDE EFFECTS AND PITFALLS

It is imperative that the clinician rules out causes of obturator neuralgia that, if undiagnosed, could harm the patient, such as uncontrolled diabetes and retroperitoneal or pelvic tumor. The main side effect of obturator nerve block is postblock ecchymosis and hematoma. The potential for needle induced trauma to the obturator nerve remains a possibility. By advancing the needle slowly and then withdrawing the needle slightly away from the nerve, needle-induced trauma to the obturator nerve can be avoided.

CLINICAL PEARLS

Obturator neuralgia should always be differentiated from lumbar plexopathy and radiculopathy of the nerve roots that may at times mimic obturator nerve compression. Furthermore, it should be remembered that lumbar radiculopathy and obturator nerve entrapment may coexist in the "double crush" syndrome. The double crush syndrome is seen most commonly with median nerve entrapment at the wrist.

Injection of the obturator nerve is a simple and safe technique in the evaluation and treatment of the above-mentioned painful conditions. Careful neurological examination to identify preexisting neurological deficits that may later be attributed to the nerve block should be performed on all patients before beginning obturator nerve block, especially in those patients with clinical symptoms of diabetes or clinically significant obturator neuralgia.

55

Saphenous Neuralgia

ICD-9 CODE 355.8

THE CLINICAL SYNDROME

Saphenous neuralgia is an uncommon cause of medial calf pain that may occur after vascular surgery on the lower extremity. With the increased number of total knee arthroplasties being performed, trauma to the infrapatellar branch of the saphenous nerve may cause damage, producing pain and numbness over the patellar tendon. Patients suffering from saphenous neuralgia often experience medial pseudoclaudication-type pain that may confuse the clinical evaluation and lead the clinician to suspect lumbar spinal stenosis. Saphenous neuralgia may also be due to compression of the nerve by tumor, hemorrhage, or abscess. This compression usually occurs at the level at which the nerve exits from Hunter's canal. Stretch injuries to the saphenous nerve can also occur at this point. Diabetes can also affect the saphenous nerve, but this is usually in conjunction with neuropathy of the other nerves of the lower extremity.

SIGNS AND SYMPTOMS

The patient with saphenous neuralgia will present with pain that radiates into the medial calf to the medial malleolus (Fig. 55–1). This pain may be paresthetic or burning in character. The intensity is moderate to severe. There is no motor deficit associated with saphenous neuropathy unless the spinal nerve roots or plexus or other peripheral nerves are involved. Patients with saphenous neuralgia may complain of a sunburned feeling over the distribution of the saphenous nerve.

TESTING

Electromyography can help identify the exact source of neurological dysfunction and help clarify the differential diagnosis and thus should be the starting point of the evaluation of all patients suspected of having saphenous neuralgia. Plain radiographs of the spine, hip, pelvis, and femur are indicated in all patients who present with saphenous neuralgia to rule out occult bony pathology. Based on the patient's clinical presentation, additional testing including complete blood cell count, uric acid, sedimentation rate, and antinuclear antibody testing may be indicated. Magnetic resonance imaging (MRI) of the spine, pelvis, and proximal lower extremity is indicated if tumor or hematoma is suspected. Injection of the saphenous nerve with a local anesthetic and steroid as it exits Hunter's canal serves as both a diagnostic and therapeutic maneuver.

DIFFERENTIAL DIAGNOSIS

It is difficult to separate saphenous neuralgia from a lumbar radiculopathy on purely clinical grounds, and electromyography is strongly recommended. Electromyography and nerve conduction testing will also help rule out the presence of peripheral neuropathy. It should be remembered that intrapelvic or retroperitoneal tumor or hematoma may compress the lumbar plexus and mimic the clinical presentation of saphenous neuralgia.

TREATMENT

Mild cases of saphenous neuralgia will usually respond to conservative therapy, and surgery should be reserved for more severe cases. Initial treatment of saphenous neuralgia should consist of treatment with simple analgesics, nonsteroidal anti-inflammatory agents, or cyclooxygenase-2 (COX-2) inhibitors and avoidance of repetitive activities that exacerbate the patient's symptomatology. If diabetes is thought to be the etiology of the patient's saphenous neuralgia, tight control of blood sugar levels is mandatory.

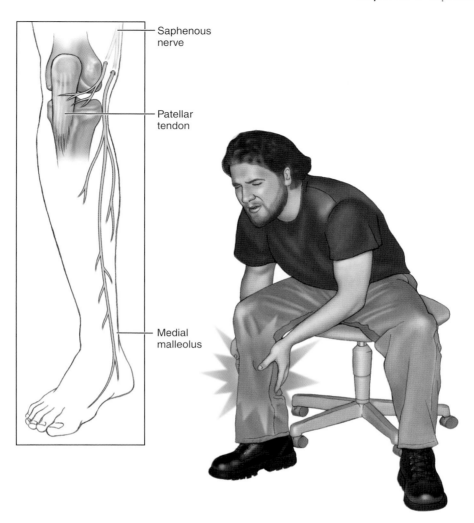

Saphenous nerve

Patellar tendon

Medial malleolus

Figure 55–1

Avoidance of repetitive activities thought to be responsible for the exacerbation of saphenous neuralgia will also help ameliorate the patient's symptoms. The use of gabapentin or a tricyclic antidepressant such as nortriptyline as an adjuvant analgesic may also help ameliorate the symptoms of saphenous neuralgia. If the patient fails to respond to these conservative measures, a next reasonable step is injection of the saphenous nerve with a local anesthetic and steroid.

SIDE EFFECTS AND PITFALLS

It is imperative that the clinician rules out causes of saphenous neuralgia that, if undiagnosed, could harm the patient, such as uncontrolled diabetes and retroperitoneal or pelvic tumor. The main side effect of saphenous nerve block is postblock ecchymosis and hematoma. The potential for needle-induced trauma to the saphenous nerve remains a possibility. By advancing the needle slowly and then withdrawing the needle slightly away from the nerve, needle-induced trauma to the saphenous nerve can be avoided.

CLINICAL PEARLS

Saphenous neuralgia should always be differentiated from lumbar plexopathy and radiculopathy of the nerve roots that may at times mimic saphenous nerve compression. Furthermore, it should be remembered that lumbar radiculopathy and saphenous nerve entrapment may coexist in the "double crush" syndrome. The double crush syndrome is seen most commonly with median nerve entrapment at the wrist.

Injection of the saphenous nerve is a simple and safe technique in the evaluation and treatment of the above-mentioned painful conditions. Careful neurological examination to identify preexisting neurological deficits that may later be attributed to the nerve block should be performed on all patients before beginning saphenous nerve block, especially in those patients with clinical symptoms of diabetes or clinically significant saphenous neuralgia.

56 Adductor Tendinitis

ICD-9 CODE 726.90

THE CLINICAL SYNDROME

The increased use of exercise equipment in gyms for lower extremity strengthening has resulted in an increased incidence of adductor tendinitis. The adductor muscles of the hip include the gracilis, adductor longus, adductor brevis, and adductor magnus muscles. The adductor function of these muscles is innervated by the obturator nerve, which is susceptible to trauma from pelvic fractures and compression by tumor. The tendons of the adductor muscles of the hip have their origin along the pubis and ischial ramus, and it is at this point that tendinitis frequently occurs.

These tendons and their associated muscles are susceptible to the development of tendinitis due to overuse or trauma due to stretch injuries. Inciting factors may include the vigorous use of exercise equipment for lower extremity strengthening and acute stretching of the musculotendinous units as a result of sports injuries, such as sliding into bases when playing baseball.

The pain of adductor tendinitis is sharp, constant, and severe, with sleep disturbance often reported. The patient may attempt to splint the inflamed tendons by adopting an adductor lurch type of gait, that is, shifting the trunk of the body over the affected extremity when walking. In addition to the above-mentioned pain, patients suffering from adductor tendinitis will often experience a gradual decrease in functional ability, with decreasing hip range of motion making simple everyday tasks such as getting in or out of an automobile quite difficult. With continued disuse, muscle wasting may occur, and an adhesive capsulitis of the hip may develop.

SIGNS AND SYMPTOMS

On physical examination, the patient suffering from adductor tendinitis will report pain on palpation of the origins of the adductor tendons. Active resisted adduction will reproduce the pain, as will passive abduction (Fig. 56–1). Tendinitis of the musculotendinous unit of the hip frequently coexists with bursitis of the associated bursae of the hip joint, creating additional pain and functional disability. Neurological examination of the hip and lower extremity will be within normal limits unless there has been concomitant stretch injury to the plexus or obturator nerve.

TESTING

Plain radiographs are indicated in all patients who present with hip, thigh, and groin pain. Based on the patient's clinical presentation, additional testing including complete blood cell count, sedimentation rate, and antinuclear antibody testing may be indicated. Magnetic resonance imaging (MRI) of the hip is indicated if aseptic necrosis or occult mass is suspected. Radionucleotide bone scanning should be considered if the possibility of occult fracture of the pelvis is being considered. Electromyography can help rule out compression neuropathy or trauma of the obturator nerve and rule out plexopathy and radiculopathy. Injection of the insertion of the adductor tendons serves as both a diagnostic and therapeutic maneuver.

DIFFERENTIAL DIAGNOSIS

Internal derangement of the hip may mimic the clinical presentation of adductor tendinitis. Occasionally, indirect inguinal hernia can produce pain that can be confused with adductor tendinitis. If trauma has occurred, consideration of the possibility

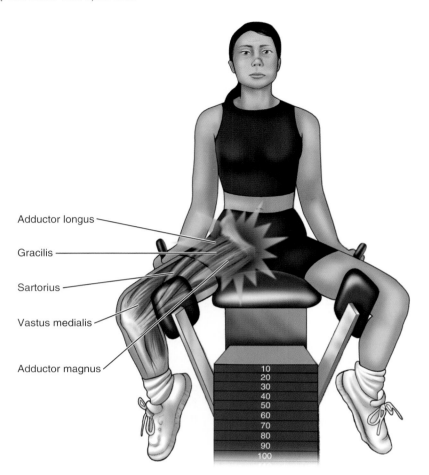

Adductor longus

Gracilis

Sartorius

Vastus medialis

Adductor magnus

Figure 56–1

of occult pelvic fracture, especially in those individuals with osteopenia or osteoporosis, should be entertained and radionucleotide bone scanning obtained. Avascular necrosis of the hip may also produce hip pain that can mimic the clinical presentation of adductor tendinitis. Entrapment neuropathy and/or stretch injury to the ilioinguinal, genitofemoral, and obturator nerves as well as plexopathy and radiculopathy should be considered if there is the physical finding of neurological deficit in those patients thought to suffer from adductor tendinitis, as all of these clinical entities may coexist.

TREATMENT

Initial treatment of the pain and functional disability associated with adductor tendinitis should include a combination of the nonsteroidal anti-inflammatory agents or cyclooxygenase-2 (COX-2) inhibitors and physical therapy. The local application of heat and cold may also be beneficial. For patients who do not respond to these treatment modalities, the injection of the insertion of the adductor tendons of the hip with a local anesthetic and steroid may be a reasonable next step.

SIDE EFFECTS AND PITFALLS

If trauma is present, the possibility of occult pelvic fracture should always be considered, as should the possibility of occult malignancy of the pelvis or hip.

The possibility of trauma to the adductor tendons from injection of the tendinous insertion remains an ever-present possibility. Tendons that are highly inflamed or previously damaged are subject to rupture if they are directly injected. This complication can be greatly decreased if the clinician uses gentle technique and stops injecting immediately if significant resistance to injection is encountered. Approximately 25% of patients will complain of a transient increase in pain after this injection technique and should be warned of such.

CLINICAL PEARLS

The proper use of exercise equipment can greatly reduce the incidence of adductor tendinitis. Injection of the adductor tendons is extremely effective in the treatment of pain secondary to the above-mentioned causes of hip pain. Gentle injection technique will decrease the incidence of traumatic rupture of the tendons due to injection. Coexistent bursitis and arthritis may also contribute to hip pain and may require additional treatment with a more localized injection of a local anesthetic and depot-steroid. The use of physical modalities, including local heat as well as gentle range of motion exercises, should be introduced several days after the patient undergoes this injection technique for hip pain. Vigorous exercises should be avoided because they will exacerbate the patient's symptomatology. Simple analgesics and nonsteroidal anti-inflammatory agents may be used concurrently with this injection technique.

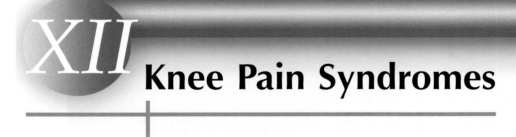

XII Knee Pain Syndromes

57 *Tibiofibular Pain Syndrome*

ICD-9 CODE 715.96

THE CLINICAL SYNDROME

Tibiofibular joint pain is most often the result of arthritis of the joint. Osteoarthritis of the joint is the most common form of arthritis that results in tibiofibular joint pain. However, rheumatoid arthritis and post-traumatic arthritis are also common causes of tibiofibular pain secondary to arthritis. The tibiofibular joint is frequently damaged from falls with the foot fully medially rotated and the knee flexed, and such trauma will frequently result in post-traumatic arthritis. Less common causes of arthritis-induced tibiofibular pain include the collagen vascular diseases, infection, villonodular synovitis, and Lyme disease. In addition to arthritis, the tibiofibular joint is susceptible to the development of tendinitis, bursitis, and disruption of the ligaments, cartilage, and tendons, all of which may cause pain and functional disability.

The majority of patients presenting with tibiofibular pain secondary to osteoarthritis and post-traumatic arthritis will present with the complaint of pain that is localized around the tibiofibular joint and the lateral aspect of the knee. Activity, especially involving flexion and medial rotation of the knee, will make the pain worse, with rest and heat providing some relief. The pain is constant and characterized as aching in nature. The pain may interfere with sleep.

SIGNS AND SYMPTOMS

Examination of the knee in patients suffering from tibiofibular joint pain will reveal tenderness to palpation of the lateral aspect of the knee. Some patients will complain of a grating or popping sensation with use of the joint and crepitus may be present on physical examination. In addition to the above-mentioned pain, patients suffering from arthritis of the tibiofibular joint will often experience a gradual decrease in functional ability with decreasing tibiofibular joint range of motion, making simple everyday tasks such as walking, climbing stairs, and getting in and out of an automobile quite difficult. Morning stiffness and stiffness after sitting for prolonged periods are common complaints of patients suffering from arthritis of the tibiofibular joint. With continued disuse, muscle weakness and wasting may occur, and loss of support from the muscles and ligaments will eventually make the tibiofibular joint unstable. This instability is most evident when the patient attempts to walk on uneven surfaces or climb stairs (Fig. 57–1).

TESTING

Plain radiographs of the knee are indicated in all patients who present with tibiofibular joint pain. Based on the patient's clinical presentation, additional testing including complete blood cell count, sedimentation rate, and antinuclear antibody testing may be indicated. Magnetic resonance imaging (MRI) of the tibiofibular joint is indicated if aseptic necrosis or occult mass or tumor is suspected. Bone scan may be useful to identify occult stress fractures involving the joint, especially if trauma has occurred.

DIFFERENTIAL DIAGNOSIS

The tibiofibular joint is susceptible to the development of arthritis from a variety of conditions that have in common the ability to damage the joint cartilage. Acute infectious arthritis will usually be accompanied by significant systemic symptoms, including fever and malaise, and should be easily recognized by the astute clinician and treated appropriately with culture and antibiotics, rather than with

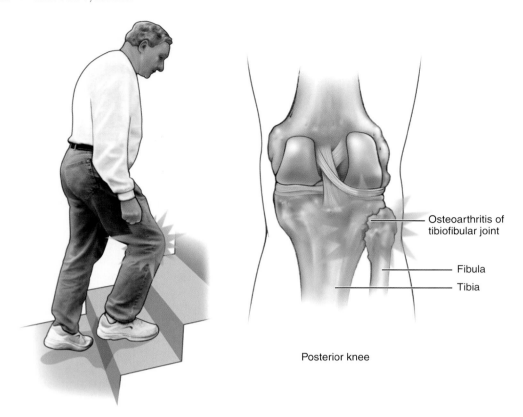

Osteoarthritis of
tibiofibular joint

Fibula

Tibia

Posterior knee

Figure 57–1

injection therapy. The collagen vascular diseases will generally present as a polyarthropathy rather than a monoarthropathy limited to the tibiofibular joint, although tibiofibular pain secondary to collagen vascular disease responds exceedingly well to the intra-articular injection technique described below. Lumbar radiculopathy may mimic the pain and disability associated with arthritis of the tibiofibular joint. In such patients, the knee examination should be negative. Entrapment neuropathies such as meralgia paresthetica may also confuse the diagnosis as may bursitis of the knee, both of which may coexist with arthritis of the tibiofibular joint. Primary and metastatic tumors of the femur and spine may also present clinically in a manner analogous to arthritis of the knee.

TREATMENT

Initial treatment of the pain and functional disability associated with arthritis of the knee should include a combination of the nonsteroidal anti-inflammatory agents or cyclooxygenase-2 (COX-2) inhibitors and physical therapy. The local application of heat and cold may also be beneficial. For patients who do not respond to these treatment modalities, an intra-articular injection of a local anesthetic and steroid may be a reasonable next step.

SIDE EFFECTS AND COMPLICATIONS

Failure to identify primary or metastatic tumor of the knee or spine that is responsible for the patient's

pain may yield disastrous results. The major complication of intra-articular injection of the knee is infection. This complication should be exceedingly rare if strict aseptic technique is adhered to. Approximately 25% of patients will complain of a transient increase in pain following intra-articular injection of the knee joint and should be warned of such.

CLINICAL PEARLS

Coexistent bursitis and tendinitis may also contribute to tibiofibular pain and may require additional treatment with more localized injection of a local anesthetic and depot-steroid. Injection of the tibiofibular joint is extremely effective in the treatment of pain secondary to the above-mentioned causes of arthritis of the knee joint. This technique is a safe procedure if careful attention is paid to the clinically relevant anatomy in the areas to be injected. Care must be taken to use sterile technique to avoid infection, as well as the use of universal precautions to avoid risk to the operator. The use of physical modalities, including local heat as well as gentle range of motion exercises, should be introduced several days after the patient undergoes this injection technique for knee pain. Vigorous exercises should be avoided because they will exacerbate the patient's symptomatology.

58 *Semimembranous Insertion Pain Syndrome*

ICD-9 CODE 719.46

THE CLINICAL SYNDROME

Semimembranous insertion pain syndrome is an uncommon cause of posterior knee pain encountered in clinical practice. Patients suffering from semimembranous insertion syndrome will exhibit localized tenderness over the posterior aspect of the medial knee joint, with severe pain being elicited on palpation of the attachment of the semimembranosus muscle at the posterior medial condyle of the tibia. The semimembranosus muscle flexes and medially rotates the leg at the knee as well as extending the thigh at the hip joint. A fibrous extension of the muscle called the *oblique popliteal ligament* extends upward and laterally to provide support to the posterior knee joint. This ligament as well as the tendinous insertion of the muscle is prone to the development of inflammation from overuse, misuse, or trauma.

Semimembranosus insertion pain syndrome occurs most commonly after overuse or misuse of the knee, often following overaggressive exercise regimens. Direct trauma to the posterior knee by kicks or tackles during football may also result in the development of semimembranosus insertion syndrome (Fig. 58–1). Coexistent inflammation of the semimembranosus bursa that lies between the medial head of the gastrocnemius muscle, the medial femoral epicondyle and the semimembranosus tendon may exacerbate the pain of semimembranosus insertion syndrome.

SIGNS AND SYMPTOMS

On physical examination, the patient suffering from semimembranous insertion pain syndrome will exhibit point tenderness over the attachment of the semimembranosus muscle at the posterior medial condyle of the tibia. The patient may be tender over the posterior knee, with pain being reproduced with passive rotation of the flexed knee with patient in the prone position. Internal derangement of the knee may also be present and should be searched for on examination of the knee, as should Baker's cyst.

TESTING

Plain radiographs are indicated in all patients who present with pain thought to be emanating from semimembranosus insertion syndrome to rule out occult bony pathology, including tibial plateau fractures and tumor. Based on the patient's clinical presentation, additional testing including complete blood cell count, prostate specific antigen, sedimentation rate, and antinuclear antibody testing may be indicated. Magnetic resonance imaging (MRI) of the knee is indicated if internal derangement, occult mass, or tumor is suspected. Radionucleotide bone scanning may be useful to rule out stress fractures not seen on plain radiographs. Injection of the semimembranous insertions with a local anesthetic and steroid serves as both a diagnostic and therapeutic maneuver.

DIFFERENTIAL DIAGNOSIS

The most common cause of posterior knee pain is due to arthritis of the knee. This should be readily identifiable on plain radiographs of the knee and may coexist with semimembranous insertion pain syndrome. Another common cause of posterior knee pain is Baker's cyst, which is a herniation of the synovial sac posteriorly into the popliteal fossa. Rarely, aneurysm of the tibial artery may cause pain that may mimic the pain of semimembranous insertion pain syndrome. As mentioned, inflammation of the semimembranous bursa may also cause posterior knee pain.

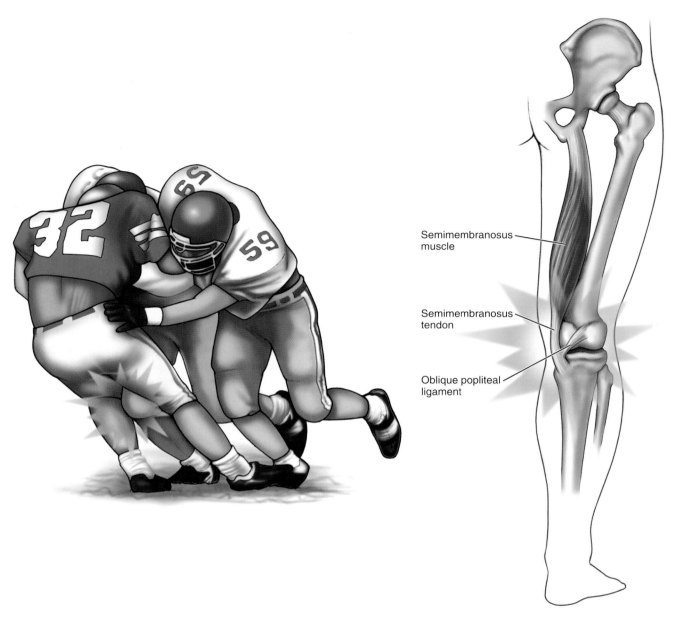

Semimembranosus muscle

Semimembranosus tendon

Oblique popliteal ligament

Figure 58–1

TREATMENT

Initial treatment of the pain and functional disability associated with semimembranous insertion pain syndrome should include a combination of the nonsteroidal anti-inflammatory agents or cyclooxygenase-2 (COX-2) inhibitors and physical therapy. The local application of heat and cold may also be beneficial. For patients who do not respond to these treatment modalities, injection of a local anesthetic and steroid may be a reasonable next step.

The goals of this injection technique are explained to the patient. The patient is placed in the prone position with the anterior ankle resting on a folded towel to slightly flex the knee. The medial condyle of the tibia is then identified and at a point 2 cm below the medial joint line is the insertion of the semimembranosus muscle. Proper preparation with antiseptic solution of the skin overlying this point is then carried out. A syringe containing 2.0 mL of 0.25% preservative-free bupivacaine and 40 mg of methylprednisolone is attached to a 25-gauge 3½-inch needle.

The needle is then carefully advanced through the previously identified point at a right angle to the skin directly toward the insertion point of the semimembranosus muscle. The needle is advanced very slowly until the needle impinges on the medial condyle of the tibia. The needle is then withdrawn slightly back out of the periosteum of the tibia. After careful aspiration for blood and if no paresthesia is present in the distribution of the common peroneal or tibial nerve, the contents of the syringe are then gently injected. There should be minimal resistance to injection.

SIDE EFFECTS AND COMPLICATIONS

Failure to identify primary or metastatic tumor of the knee or spine that is responsible for the patient's pain may yield disastrous results. The major complication of injection of the semimembranous insertion is infection. This complication should be exceedingly rare if strict aseptic technique is adhered to. Approximately 25% of patients will complain of a transient increase in pain after injection of the semimembranous insertion and should be warned of such.

CLINICAL PEARLS

Coexistent bursitis and arthritis may also contribute to the pain of semimembranous insertion pain syndrome and may require additional treatment with more localized injection of a local anesthetic and depot-steroid. Injection of the semimembranous insertion is extremely effective in the treatment of pain secondary to this painful condition. This technique is a safe procedure if careful attention is paid to the clinically relevant anatomy in the areas to be injected. Care must be taken to use sterile technique to avoid infection, as well as the use of universal precautions to avoid risk to the operator. The use of physical modalities, including local heat as well as gentle range of motion exercises, should be introduced several days after the patient undergoes this injection technique for knee pain. Vigorous exercises should be avoided because they will exacerbate the patient's symptomatology.

59 *Quadriceps Expansion Syndrome*

ICD-9 CODE 727.09

THE CLINICAL SYNDROME

The quadriceps expansion syndrome is an uncommon cause of anterior knee pain encountered in clinical practice. This painful condition is characterized by pain at the superior pole of the patella. It is usually the result of overuse or misuse of the knee joint such as running marathons or direct trauma to the quadriceps tendon from a kick or head butts during football. The quadriceps tendon is also subject to acute calcific tendinitis, which may coexist with acute strain injuries. Calcific tendinitis of the quadriceps tendon will have a characteristic radiographic appearance of whiskers on the anterosuperior patella.

The quadriceps tendon is made up of fibers from the four muscles that compose the quadriceps muscle: the vastus lateralis, the vastus intermedius, the vastus medialis, and the rectus femoris. Fibers of the quadriceps tendon expanding around the patella form the medial and lateral patella retinacula and help strengthen the knee joint. These fibers are called *expansions* and are subject to strain, and the tendon proper is subject to the development of tendinitis.

Patients with quadriceps expansion syndrome will present with pain over the superior pole of the patella, more commonly on the medial side. The patient will note increased pain on walking down slopes or down stairs (Fig. 59–1). Activity involving the knee will make the pain worse, with rest and heat providing some relief. The pain is constant and characterized as aching in nature. The pain may interfere with sleep.

SIGNS AND SYMPTOMS

On physical examination, patients suffering from quadriceps expansion syndrome will have tenderness under the superior edge of the patella, occurring more commonly on the medial side. Active resisted extension of the knee will reproduce the pain. Coexistent suprapatellar and infrapatellar bursitis, tendinitis, arthritis, and/or internal derangement of the knee may confuse the clinical picture following trauma to the knee joint.

TESTING

Plain radiographs of the knee are indicated in all patients who present with quadriceps expansion syndrome pain. Based on the patient's clinical presentation, additional testing including complete blood cell count, sedimentation rate, and antinuclear antibody testing may be indicated. Magnetic resonance imaging (MRI) of the knee is indicated if internal derangement or occult mass or tumor is suspected. Bone scan may be useful to identify occult stress fractures involving the joint, especially if trauma has occurred.

DIFFERENTIAL DIAGNOSIS

The most common cause of anterior knee pain is due to arthritis of the knee. This should be readily identifiable on plain radiographs of the knee and may coexist with quadriceps expansion syndrome. Another common cause of anterior knee pain that may mimic or coexist with quadriceps expansion syndrome is suprapatellar or prepatellar bursitis. Internal derangement of the knee or torn medial meniscus may also confuse the clinical diagnosis but should be readily identifiable on MRI of the knee.

TREATMENT

Initial treatment of the pain and functional disability associated with quadriceps expansion syndrome should include a combination of the nonsteroidal

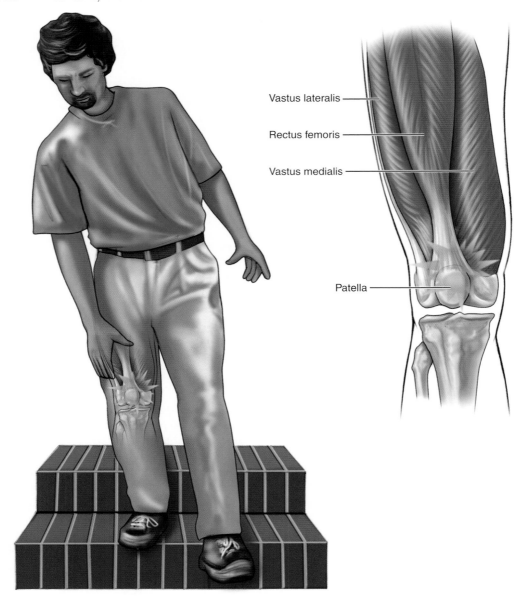

Vastus lateralis

Rectus femoris

Vastus medialis

Patella

Figure 59–1

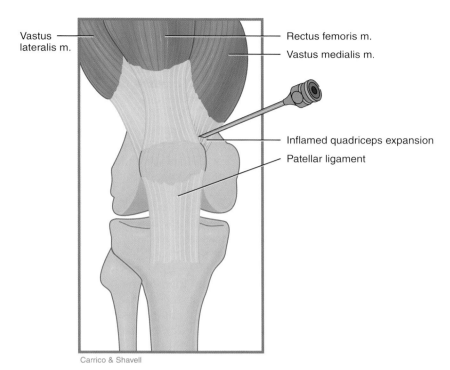

Vastus lateralis m.

Rectus femoris m.

Vastus medialis m.

Inflamed quadriceps expansion

Patellar ligament

Carrico & Shavell

Figure 59–2. (From Waldman SD: Atlas of Pain Management Injection Techniques. Philadelphia, WB Saunders, 2000, p 266.)

anti-inflammatory agents or cyclooxygenase-2 (COX-2) inhibitors and physical therapy. The local application of heat and cold may also be beneficial. For patients who do not respond to these treatment modalities, injection of the quadriceps expansion with a local anesthetic and steroid may be a reasonable next step.

To inject the quadriceps expansion, the patient is placed in the supine position with a rolled blanket underneath the knee to gently flex the joint. The skin overlying the medial aspect of the knee joint is prepped with antiseptic solution. A sterile syringe containing 2.0 mL of 0.25% preservative-free bupivacaine and 40 mg of methylprednisolone is attached to a 25-gauge 1½-inch needle using strict aseptic technique. With strict aseptic technique, the medial edge of the superior patella is identified (Fig. 59–2). At this point, the needle is inserted horizontally toward the medial edge of the patella. The needle is then carefully advanced through the skin and subcutaneous tissues until it impinges on the medial edge of the patella. The needle is then withdrawn slightly out of the periosteum of the patella, and the contents of the syringe are then gently injected. There should be little resistance to injection. If resistance is encountered, the needle is probably in a ligament or tendon and should be advanced or withdrawn slightly until the injection proceeds without significant resistance. The needle is then removed, and a sterile pressure dressing and ice pack are placed at the injection site.

SIDE EFFECTS AND PITFALLS

The major complication of this injection technique is infection. This complication should be exceedingly rare if strict aseptic technique is adhered to. Approximately 25% of patients will complain of a transient increase in pain after injection of the quadriceps tendon of the knee and should be warned of such. The clinician should also identify coexistent internal derangement of the knee, primary and metastatic tumors, and infection, which, if undiagnosed, may yield disastrous results.

CLINICAL PEARLS

This injection technique is extremely effective in the treatment of pain secondary to the causes of quadriceps extension syndrome mentioned earlier. Coexistent bursitis, tendinitis, arthritis, and internal derangement of the knee may also contribute to the patient's pain and may require additional treatment with more localized injection of a local anesthetic and depot-steroid. This technique is a safe procedure if careful attention is paid to the clinically relevant anatomy in the areas to be injected. Care must be taken to use sterile technique to avoid infection, as well as the use of universal precautions to avoid risk to the operator. The use of physical modalities, including local heat as well as gentle range of motion exercises, should be introduced several days after the patient undergoes this injection technique for tibiofibular pain. Vigorous exercises should be avoided because they will exacerbate the patient's symptomatology. Simple analgesics and nonsteroidal anti-inflammatory agents may be used concurrently with this injection technique.

60 *Coronary Ligament Strain*

ICD-9 CODE 844.8

THE CLINICAL SYNDROME

An often-overlooked cause of medial knee pain, strain of the coronary ligaments can cause significant pain and functional disability. The coronary ligaments are thin bands of fibrous tissue that anchor the medial meniscus to the tibial plateau. The coronary ligaments are actually extensions of the joint capsule. These ligaments are susceptible to disruption due to trauma from forced rotation of the knee. The medial portion of the ligament is most commonly damaged.

Patients with coronary ligament syndrome will present with pain over the medial joint and increased pain on passive external rotation of the knee. Activity, especially involving flexion and external rotation of the knee, will make the pain worse (Fig. 60–1), with rest and heat providing some relief. The pain is constant and characterized as aching in nature. The pain may interfere with sleep. Coexistent bursitis, tendinitis, arthritis, and/or internal derangement of the knee, in particular of the medial meniscus, may confuse the clinical picture following trauma to the knee joint.

SIGNS AND SYMPTOMS

Patients suffering from coronary ligament strain will invariably present with a history of a rotation injury to the knee. On physical examination, the patient will exhibit medial joint tenderness and a marked increase in pain with passive external rotation of the knee. A joint effusion may be present. Subtle knee instability will be hard to detect on physical examination due to splinting of the knee as a result of the amount of pain associated with this injury. The neurological examination of the patient suffering from coronary ligament strain is within normal limits. As

mentioned, coexistent bursitis, tendinitis, arthritis, and/or internal derangement of the knee, in particular of the medial meniscus, may make a diagnosis on a purely clinical basis difficult to make.

TESTING

Plain radiographs are indicated in all patients who present with coronary ligament syndrome pain. Based on the patient's clinical presentation, additional testing including complete blood cell count, sedimentation rate, and antinuclear antibody testing may be indicated. Magnetic resonance imaging (MRI) of the knee is indicated to quantify the extent of internal derangement of the knee and to rule out occult mass or tumor. Bone scan may be useful to identify occult stress fractures involving the joint, especially if significant trauma has occurred.

DIFFERENTIAL DIAGNOSIS

The most common cause of medial knee pain is degenerative arthritis of the knee. However, other pathological processes may mimic the pain and functional disability of coronary ligament strain. Lumbar radiculopathy may cause pain and disability similar to that of coronary ligament strain. In such patients, back pain is usually present and the knee examination should be negative. Entrapment neuropathies of the lower extremity such as femoral neuropathy may also confuse the diagnosis, as may bursitis of the knee, both of which may coexist with coronary ligament strain. Primary and metastatic tumors of the femur and spine may also present in a manner analogous to coronary ligament strain.

TREATMENT

Initial treatment of the pain and functional disability associated with coronary ligament strain should

219

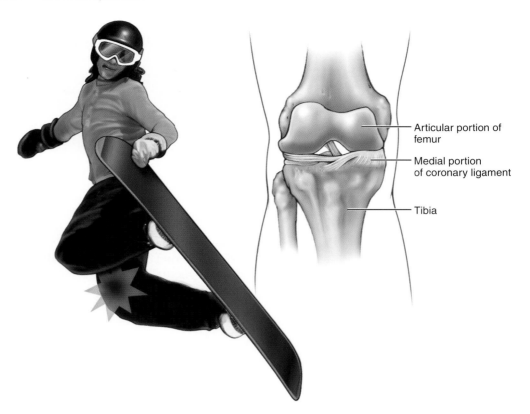

Articular portion of femur

Medial portion of coronary ligament

Tibia

Figure 60–1

include a combination of the nonsteroidal anti-inflammatory agents or cyclooxygenase-2 (COX-2) inhibitors and physical therapy. The local application of heat and cold may also be beneficial. For patients who do not respond to these treatment modalities, injection of the coronary ligament with a local anesthetic and steroid may be a reasonable next step.

SIDE EFFECTS AND PITFALLS

Failure to identify primary or metastatic tumor of the knee or spine that is responsible for the patient's pain may yield disastrous results. The major complication of injection of the coronary ligament is infection. This complication should be exceedingly rare if strict aseptic technique is adhered to. Approximately 25% of patients will complain of a transient increase in pain after injection of the coronary ligament and should be warned of such.

CLINICAL PEARLS

Coexistent bursitis and tendinitis may also contribute to knee pain and may require additional treatment with more localized injection of a local anesthetic and depot-steroid. Injection of the coronary ligament is extremely effective in the treatment of pain secondary to coronary ligament strain. This technique is a safe procedure if careful attention is paid to the clinically relevant anatomy in the areas to be injected. The use of physical modalities, including local heat as well as gentle range of motion exercises, should be introduced several days after the patient undergoes this injection technique for knee pain. Vigorous exercises should be avoided because they will exacerbate the patient's symptomatology.

61 *Iliotibial Band Bursitis*

ICD-9 CODE 726.60

THE CLINICAL SYNDROME

With the increased interest in jogging and long distance bicycling, iliotibial band bursitis is being encountered more frequently in clinical practice. The iliotibial band bursa lies between the iliotibial band and the lateral condyle of the femur. The iliotibial band is an extension of the fascia lata, which inserts at the lateral condyle of the tibia. The iliotibial band can rub back and forth over the lateral epicondyle of the femur and irritate the iliotibial bursa beneath it.

Patients with iliotibial band bursitis will present with pain over the lateral side of the distal femur just over the lateral femoral condyle. The onset of iliotibial bursitis frequently occurs after long distance biking or jogging with worn-out shoes without proper cushioning. Activity, especially involving resisted abduction and passive adduction of the lower extremity, will make the pain worse, with rest and heat providing some relief. Flexion of the affected knee will also reproduce the pain in many patients suffering from iliotibial band bursitis. Often, the patient will be unable to kneel or walk down stairs (Fig. 61–1). The pain is constant and characterized as aching in nature. The pain may interfere with sleep. Coexistent bursitis, tendinitis, arthritis, and/or internal derangement of the knee may confuse the clinical picture after trauma to the knee joint. If the inflammation of the iliotibial band bursae becomes chronic, calcification of the bursae may occur.

SIGNS AND SYMPTOMS

Physical examination may reveal point tenderness over the lateral condyle of the femur just above the tendinous insertion of the iliotibial band. Swelling and fluid accumulation surrounding the bursa is often present. Palpation of this area while having the patient flex and extend the knee may result in a creaking or catching sensation. Active resisted abduction of the lower extremity will reproduce the pain as will passive adduction. Sudden release of resistance during this maneuver will markedly increase the pain. Pain will be exacerbated by having the patient stand with all weight on the affected extremity and then flexing the affected knee 30–40 degrees.

TESTING

Plain radiographs of the knee may reveal calcification of the bursa and associated structures, including the iliotibial band tendon, consistent with chronic inflammation. Magnetic resonance imaging (MRI) is indicated if internal derangement, occult mass, or tumor of the knee is suspected. If arthritis is suspected, screening laboratory tests including a complete blood cell count, sedimentation rate, automated chemistries, and antinuclear antibody testing should be obtained. Electromyography will help distinguish iliotibial band bursitis from neuropathy, lumbar radiculopathy, and plexopathy. The following injection technique serves as a diagnostic and therapeutic maneuver.

DIFFERENTIAL DIAGNOSIS

The most common cause of lateral knee pain is degenerative arthritis of the knee. However, other pathological processes may mimic the pain and functional disability of iliotibial band bursitis. Lumbar radiculopathy may cause pain and disability similar to that of iliotibial band bursitis. In such patients, back pain is usually present, and the knee examination should be negative. Entrapment neuropathies of the lower extremity such as meralgia paresthetica may also confuse the diagnosis as may bursitis of the

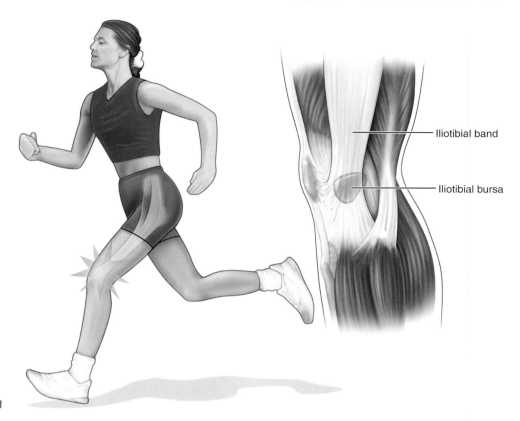

Figure 61–1

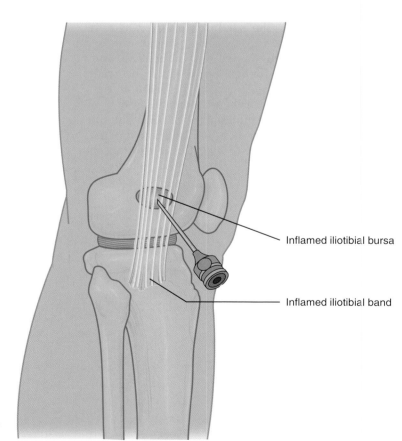

Figure 61–2. (From Waldman SD: Atlas of Pain Management Injection Techniques. Philadelphia, WB Saunders, 2000, p 283.)

knee, both of which may coexist with iliotibial band bursitis. Primary and metastatic tumors of the femur and spine may also present in a manner analogous to iliotibial band bursitis.

TREATMENT

Initial treatment of the pain and functional disability associated with iliotibial band bursitis should include a combination of the nonsteroidal anti-inflammatory agents or cyclooxygenase-2 (COX-2) inhibitors and physical therapy. The local application of heat and cold may also be beneficial. For patients who do not respond to these treatment modalities, injection of the iliotibial band bursa with a local anesthetic and steroid may be a reasonable next step.

The iliotibial band bursa is injected by placing the patient in the supine position with a rolled blanket underneath the knee to gently flex the joint. The skin over the lateral epicondyle of the femur is prepped with antiseptic solution. A sterile syringe containing 2.0 mL of 0.25% preservative-free bupivacaine and 40 mg of methylprednisolone is attached to a 25-gauge 1½-inch needle using strict aseptic technique. With strict aseptic technique, the iliotibial band bursa is located by identifying the point of maximal tenderness over the lateral condyle of the femur. The bursa will usually be identified by point tenderness at that spot. At this point, the needle is inserted at a 45-degree angle to the femoral condyle to pass through the skin, subcutaneous tissues, and the iliotibial band into the iliotibial band bursa (Fig. 61–2). If the needle strikes the femur, it is the withdrawn slightly into the substance of the bursa. When the needle is in position in proximity to the iliotibial band bursa, the contents of the syringe are then gently injected. There should be little resistance to injection. If resistance is

encountered, the needle is probably in a ligament or tendon and should be advanced or withdrawn slightly until the injection proceeds without significant resistance. The needle is then removed, and a sterile pressure dressing and ice pack are placed at the injection site.

SIDE EFFECTS AND PITFALLS

Failure to identify primary or metastatic tumor of the knee or spine that is responsible for the patient's pain may yield disastrous results. The major complication of injection of the iliotibial band bursa is infection. This complication should be exceedingly rare if strict aseptic technique is adhered to. Approximately 25% of patients will complain of a transient increase in pain after injection of the iliotibial band bursa and should be warned of such.

CLINICAL PEARLS

Coexistent bursitis and tendinitis may also contribute to knee pain and may require additional treatment with more localized injection of a local anesthetic and depot-steroid. Injection of the iliotibial band bursa is extremely effective in the treatment of pain secondary to iliotibial band bursitis. This technique is a safe procedure if careful attention is paid to the clinically relevant anatomy in the areas to be injected. The use of physical modalities, including local heat as well as gentle range of motion exercises, should be introduced several days after the patient undergoes this injection technique for knee pain. Vigorous exercises should be avoided because they will exacerbate the patient's symptomatology.

62 *Hamstring Tendinitis*

ICD-9 CODE 727.00

THE CLINICAL SYNDROME

Hamstring tendinitis is occurring with greater frequency owing to the increased interest in jogging and the use of exercise equipment for lower extremity strengthening. The onset of hamstring tendinitis is usually acute, occurring after overuse or misuse of the muscle group. Inciting factors may include long distance running, dancing injuries, or the vigorous use of exercise equipment for lower extremity strengthening. The pain will be constant and severe, with sleep disturbance often reported. The patient may attempt to splint the inflamed tendon by holding the knee in a slightly flexed position and assuming a lurch-type antalgic gait. In addition to the pain mentioned, patients suffering from hamstring tendinitis will often experience a gradual decrease in functional ability with decreasing knee range of motion, making simple everyday tasks such as walking, climbing stairs, or getting into an automobile quite difficult. With continued disuse, muscle wasting may occur, and a stiff knee may develop.

SIGNS AND SYMPTOMS

Patients with hamstring tendinitis will exhibit severe pain to palpation over the tendinous insertion, with the medial portion of the tendon more commonly affected than the lateral portion (Fig. 62–1). Crepitus or a creaking sensation may be felt when palpating the tendon while the patient flexes the affected knee. No mass in the popliteal fossa will be present as is seen with Baker's cyst. The neurological examination of the patient suffering from hamstring tendinitis is within normal limits.

TESTING

Plain radiographs are indicated in all patients who present with posterior knee pain. Based on the patient's clinical presentation, additional testing including complete blood cell count, sedimentation rate, and antinuclear antibody testing may be indicated. Magnetic resonance imaging (MRI) of the knee is indicated if internal derangement, occult mass, Baker's cyst, or partial tendon disruption is suspected. Injection of the hamstring tendons serves as both a diagnostic and therapeutic maneuver.

DIFFERENTIAL DIAGNOSIS

The most common cause of posterior joint pain is a Baker's cyst. Baker's cyst is a herniation of the synovial sac of the knee. Baker's cyst may rupture spontaneously and may be misdiagnosed as thrombophlebitis. Occasionally, injury to the medial meniscus may be confused with hamstring tendinitis. Primary or metastatic tumors in the region, although rare, must be considered in the differential diagnosis.

TREATMENT

Initial treatment of the pain and functional disability associated with hamstring tendinitis should include a combination of the nonsteroidal anti-inflammatory agents or cyclooxygenase-2 (COX-2) inhibitors and physical therapy. The local application of heat and cold may also be beneficial. Patients with hamstring tendinitis should avoid the repetitive activities responsible for the development of this painful condition. For patients who do not respond to these treatment modalities, injection of the hamstring tendons with a local anesthetic and steroid may be a reasonable next step.

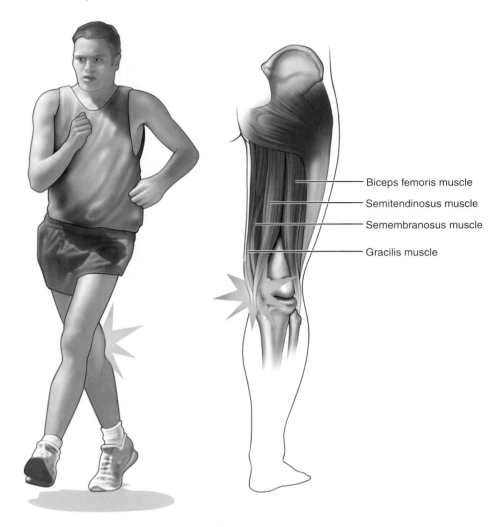

Biceps femoris muscle
Semitendinosus muscle
Semembranosus muscle
Gracilis muscle

Figure 62–1

SIDE EFFECTS AND PITFALLS

Failure to diagnose primary knee pathology (e.g., tears of the medial meniscus) may lead to further pain and disability. MRI should help identify internal derangement of the knee. The possibility of trauma to the hamstring tendon from the injection itself remains an ever-present possibility. Tendons that are highly inflamed or previously damaged are subject to rupture if they are directly injected. This complication can be greatly decreased if the clinician uses gentle technique and stops injecting immediately if significant resistance to injection is encountered. The proximity to the common peroneal and tibial nerve as well as the popliteal artery and vein makes it imperative that this procedure be carried out only by those well versed in the regional anatomy and experienced in performing injection techniques. Many patients will also complain of a transient increase in pain after the injection technique mentioned. Although rare, infection may occur if careful attention to sterile technique is not followed.

CLINICAL PEARLS

The musculotendinous insertion of the hamstring group of muscles is susceptible to the development of tendinitis for two reasons. First, the knee joint is subjected to significant repetitive motion under weight-bearing conditions. Second, the blood supply to the musculotendinous unit is poor, making healing of microtrauma difficult. Calcium deposition around the tendon may occur if the inflammation continues, complicating subsequent treatment. Tendinitis of the musculotendinous insertion of the hamstring frequently coexists with bursitis of the associated bursae of the knee joint, creating additional pain and functional disability.

This injection technique is extremely effective in the treatment of pain secondary to the hamstring tendinitis. Coexistent bursitis and arthritis may also contribute to knee pain and may require additional treatment with a more localized injection of a local anesthetic and depot-steroid. This technique is a safe procedure if careful attention is paid to the clinically relevant anatomy in the areas to be injected. The use of physical modalities, including local heat as well as gentle range of motion exercises, should be introduced several days after the patient undergoes this injection technique. Vigorous exercises should be avoided because they will exacerbate the patient's symptomatology.

Pes Anserine Bursitis

ICD-9 CODE 726.61

THE CLINICAL SYNDROME

Less common than prepatellar and infrapatellar bursitis, pes anserine bursitis can nevertheless cause significant knee pain and functional disability. The pes anserine bursa lies between the combined tendinous insertion of the sartorius, gracilis, and semitendinosus muscles and the medial tibia. Patients with pes anserine bursitis will present with pain over the medial knee joint and increased pain on passive valgus and external rotation of the knee. Activity, especially involving flexion and external rotation of the knee, will make the pain worse, with rest and heat providing some relief. Often, the patient will be unable to kneel or walk down stairs (Fig. 63–1). The pain is constant and characterized as aching in nature. The pain may interfere with sleep. Coexistent prepatellar or infrapatellar bursitis, tendinitis, arthritis, and/or internal derangement of the knee may confuse the clinical picture after trauma to the knee joint. Frequently, the medial collateral ligament is also involved if the patient has sustained trauma to the medial knee joint. If the inflammation of the pes anserine bursae becomes chronic, calcification of the bursae may occur.

SIGNS AND SYMPTOMS

Physical examination may reveal point tenderness in the anterior knee just below the medial knee joint at the tendinous insertion of the pes anserine. Swelling and fluid accumulation surrounding the bursa are often present. Active resisted flexion of the knee will reproduce the pain. Sudden release of resistance during this maneuver will markedly increase the pain. Rarely, the pes anserine bursa will become infected in a manner analogous to infection of the prepatellar bursa.

TESTING

Plain radiographs are indicated in all patients thought to be suffering from pes anserine bursitis. Based on the patient's clinical presentation, additional testing including complete blood cell count, sedimentation rate, and antinuclear antibody testing may be indicated. Magnetic resonance imaging (MRI) of the knee is indicated to quantify the extent of internal derangement of the knee and to rule out occult mass or tumor (Fig. 63–2). Bone scan may be useful to identify occult stress fractures involving the joint, especially if significant trauma has occurred.

DIFFERENTIAL DIAGNOSIS

The most common cause of medial knee pain is degenerative arthritis of the knee. However, other pathological processes may mimic the pain and functional disability of pes anserine bursitis. Lumbar radiculopathy may cause pain and disability similar to that of pes anserine bursitis. In such patients, back pain is usually present and the knee examination should be negative. Coronary ligament strain and bursitis of other bursa of the knee may also cause medial knee pain. Entrapment neuropathies of the lower extremity such as femoral neuropathy may also confuse the diagnosis that may coexist with pes anserine bursitis. Primary and metastatic tumors of the femur and spine may also present in a manner analogous to pes anserine bursitis.

TREATMENT

Initial treatment of the pain and functional disability associated with pes anserine bursitis should include a combination of the nonsteroidal anti-

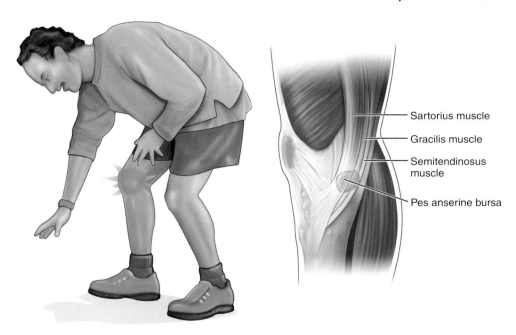

Figure 63–1

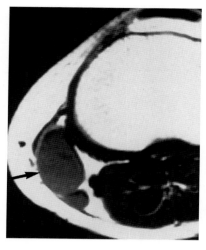

Figure 63–2. Pes anserine bursitis. T2-weighted image (SE2000/20) depicts abnormal liquid collection as a high–signal intensity region (*arrow*) seen in the axial plane. (From Stark DD, Bradley WG Jr: Magnetic Resonance Imaging, 3rd ed. St Louis, Mosby, 1999, p 857.)

inflammatory agents or cyclooxygenase-2 (COX-2) inhibitors and physical therapy. The local application of heat and cold may also be beneficial. Avoidance of the repetitive activities responsible for the evolution of this painful condition should also be considered. For patients who do not respond to these treatment modalities, injection of the coronary pes anserine bursa with a local anesthetic and steroid may be a reasonable next step.

SIDE EFFECTS AND PITFALLS

Failure to identify primary or metastatic tumor of the knee or spine that is responsible for the patient's pain may yield disastrous results. The major complication of injection of the pes anserine bursa is infection. This complication should be exceedingly rare if strict aseptic technique is adhered to. Approximately 25% of patients will complain of a transient increase in pain after injection of the pes anserine bursa and should be warned of such.

CLINICAL PEARLS

Coexistent bursitis, tendinitis, arthritis, and internal derangement of the knee may also contribute to the patient's pain and may require additional treatment with more localized injection of a local anesthetic and depot-steroid. Injection of the pes anserine bursa is extremely effective in the treatment of pain secondary to pes anserine bursitis. This technique is a safe procedure if careful attention is paid to the clinically relevant anatomy in the areas to be injected. The use of physical modalities, including local heat as well as gentle range of motion exercises, should be introduced several days after the patient undergoes this injection technique for prepatellar bursitis pain. Vigorous exercises should be avoided because it will exacerbate the patient's symptomatology. Simple analgesics and nonsteroidal anti-inflammatory agents may be used concurrently with this injection technique.

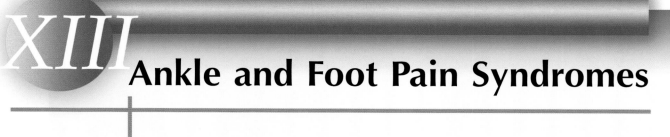

XIII Ankle and Foot Pain Syndromes

64 Subtalar Joint Pain

ICD-9 CODE 715.97

THE CLINICAL SYNDROME

Ankle and heel pain emanating from the subtalar joint is occasionally encountered in clinical practice. The subtalar joint is a synovial plane–type articulation between the talus and calcaneus. Osteoarthritis of the subtalar joint is the most common form of arthritis that results in subtalar joint pain, although the joint is also susceptible to damage from rheumatoid and post-traumatic arthritis.

The majority of patients presenting with subtalar joint pain secondary to osteoarthritis and post-traumatic arthritis pain will present with the complaint of pain that is localized deep within the heel, with a secondary dull aching pain in the ankle (Fig. 64–1). Activity, especially adduction of the calcaneus, makes the pain worse, with rest and heat providing some relief. The pain is constant and characterized as aching in nature. The pain may interfere with sleep. Some patients will complain of a grating or popping sensation with use of the joint, and crepitus may be present on physical examination.

In addition to the pain mentioned, patients suffering from arthritis of the subtalar joint will often experience a gradual decrease in functional ability with decreasing subtalar range of motion, making simple everyday tasks such as walking and climbing stairs quite difficult. With continued disuse, muscle wasting may occur and a "frozen subtalar joint" due to adhesive capsulitis may develop.

SIGNS AND SYMPTOMS

Examination of the ankle of patients suffering from arthritis of the subtalar joint will reveal diffuse tenderness to palpation. The ankle may feel hot to the touch and swelling may be present. Adduction of the calcaneus will exacerbate the pain, as will range of motion of the ankle. Weight bearing may also exacerbate the patient's pain, and a hesitant, antalgic gait may be present. Crepitus may be present on range of motion of the joint.

TESTING

Plain radiographs are indicated in all patients who present with subtalar joint pain. Based on the patient's clinical presentation, additional testing including complete blood cell count, sedimentation rate, and antinuclear antibody testing may be indicated. Magnetic resonance imaging (MRI) of the subtalar joint is indicated if joint instability, occult mass, or tumor is suspected.

DIFFERENTIAL DIAGNOSIS

The subtalar joint is susceptible to the development of arthritis from a variety of conditions that have in common the ability to damage the joint cartilage. Osteoarthritis is the most common cause, but rheumatoid arthritis and post-traumatic arthritis cause subtalar pain secondary to arthritis. Less common causes of arthritis-induced subtalar pain include the collagen vascular diseases, infection, and Lyme disease. Acute infectious arthritis will usually be accompanied by significant systemic symptoms, including fever and malaise, and should be easily recognized by the astute clinician and treated appropriately with culture and antibiotics, rather than with injection therapy. The collagen vascular diseases will generally present as a polyarthropathy rather than a monoarthropathy limited to the subtalar joint, although subtalar pain secondary to collagen vascular disease responds exceedingly well to the intra-articular injection technique described below.

Lumbar radiculopathy may mimic the pain and disability associated with arthritis of the subtalar joint. In such patients, the ankle examination should

233

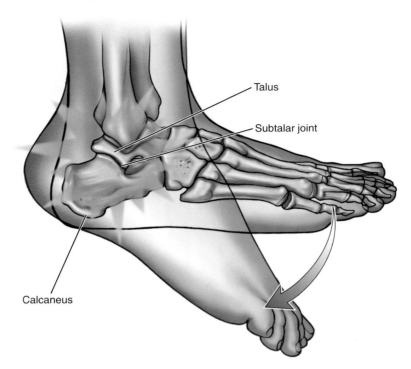

Talus

Subtalar joint

Calcaneus

Figure 64–1

be negative. Entrapment neuropathies such as tarsal tunnel syndrome may also confuse the diagnosis, as may bursitis of the ankle, both of which may coexist with arthritis of the subtalar joint. Primary and metastatic tumors of the distal tibia and fibula and spine may also present in a manner analogous to arthritis of the subtalar joint, as can occult fractures.

TREATMENT

Initial treatment of the pain and functional disability associated with arthritis of the subtalar joint should include a combination of the nonsteroidal anti-inflammatory agents or cyclooxygenase-2 (COX-2) inhibitors and physical therapy. The local application of heat and cold may also be beneficial. Avoidance of repetitive activities that aggravate the patient's symptomatology as well as short-term immobilization of the ankle joint may also provide relief. For patients who do not respond to these treatment modalities, an intra-articular injection of the subtalar joint with a local anesthetic and steroid may be a reasonable next step.

SIDE EFFECTS AND PITFALLS

Failure to identify primary or metastatic tumor of the ankle or spine that is responsible for the patient's

pain may yield disastrous results. The major complication of intra-articular injection of the subtalar joint is infection. This complication should be exceedingly rare if strict aseptic technique is adhered to. Approximately 25% of patients will complain of a transient increase in pain after intra-articular injection of the subtalar joint and should be warned of such.

CLINICAL PEARLS

Coexistent bursitis and tendinitis may also contribute to ankle pain and may require additional treatment with more localized injection of a local anesthetic and depot-steroid. The injection of the subtalar joint is extremely effective in the treatment of pain secondary to the causes of arthritis of the joint mentioned. This technique is a safe procedure if careful attention is paid to the clinically relevant anatomy in the areas to be injected. The use of physical modalities, including local heat as well as gentle range of motion exercises, should be introduced several days after the patient undergoes this injection technique for ankle pain. Vigorous exercises should be avoided because they will exacerbate the patient's symptomatology.

65 Midtarsal Joint Pain

ICD-9 CODE 715.97

THE CLINICAL SYNDROME

The midtarsal joints are an uncommon cause of ankle and foot pain. Midtarsal joint pain may be seen in patients who repeatedly point their toes, such as ballet dancers and football punters (Fig. 65–1). The majority of patients presenting with midtarsal joint pain secondary to osteoarthritis and posttraumatic arthritis pain will present with the complaint of pain that is localized to the dorsum of the foot. The muscles associated with the midtarsal joints and their attaching tendons are also susceptible to trauma and to wear and tear from overuse and misuse and may contribute to the patient's clinical symptomatology. Activity, especially inversion and adduction of the midtarsal joints, makes the pain worse, with rest and heat providing some relief. The pain is constant and characterized as aching in nature. The pain may interfere with sleep. Some patients will complain of a grating or popping sensation with use of the joint, and crepitus may be present on physical examination. In addition to the pain mentioned, patients suffering from arthritis of the midtarsal joint will often experience a gradual decrease in functional ability with decreasing midtarsal range of motion, making simple everyday tasks such as walking and climbing stairs quite difficult.

SIGNS AND SYMPTOMS

Examination of the ankle and foot of patients suffering from arthritis of the midtarsal joints will reveal diffuse tenderness to palpation. The ankle and dorsum of the foot may feel hot to touch, and swelling may be present. Adduction and inversion of the foot will exacerbate the pain, as will range of motion of the ankle. Weight bearing may also exacerbate the patient's pain, and a hesitant, antalgic gait may be present. Crepitus is often present on range of motion of the joint.

TESTING

Plain radiographs are indicated in all patients who present with midtarsal joint pain. Based on the patient's clinical presentation, additional testing including complete blood cell count, sedimentation rate, and antinuclear antibody testing may be indicated. Magnetic resonance imaging (MRI) of the midtarsal is indicated if joint instability, occult mass or tumor is suspected.

DIFFERENTIAL DIAGNOSIS

The midtarsal joint is susceptible to the development of arthritis from a variety of conditions that have in common the ability to damage the joint cartilage. Osteoarthritis of the joint is the most common form of arthritis that results in midtarsal joint pain. However, rheumatoid arthritis and posttraumatic arthritis are also common causes of midtarsal pain secondary to arthritis. Less common causes of arthritis-induced midtarsal pain include the collagen vascular diseases, infection, and Lyme disease. Acute infectious arthritis will usually be accompanied by significant systemic symptoms, including fever and malaise, and should be easily recognized by the astute clinician and treated appropriately with culture and antibiotics, rather than injection therapy. The collagen vascular diseases will generally present as a polyarthropathy rather than as a monoarthropathy limited to the midtarsal joint, although midtarsal pain secondary to collagen vascular disease responds exceedingly well to the injection of the joints with a local anesthetic and steroid.

Lumbar radiculopathy may mimic the pain and disability associated with arthritis of the midtarsal

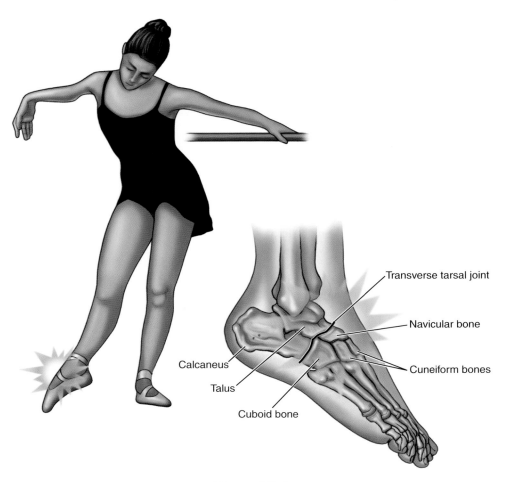

Figure 65–1

joints. In such patients, the ankle examination should be negative. Entrapment neuropathies such as tarsal tunnel syndrome may also confuse the diagnosis, as may bursitis of the ankle, both of which may coexist with arthritis of the midtarsal joint. Primary and metastatic tumors of the distal tibia and fibula and spine may also present in a manner analogous to arthritis of the midtarsal joint, as can occult fractures.

TREATMENT

Initial treatment of the pain and functional disability associated with arthritis of the midtarsal joints should include a combination of the nonsteroidal anti-inflammatory agents or cyclooxygenase-2 (COX-2) inhibitors and physical therapy. The local application of heat and cold may also be beneficial. Avoidance of repetitive activities that aggravate the patient's symptomatology as well as short-term immobilization of the ankle joint may also provide relief. For patients who do not respond to these treatment modalities, an injection of the midtarsal joints with a local anesthetic and steroid may be a reasonable next step.

SIDE EFFECTS AND PITFALLS

Failure to identify primary or metastatic tumor of the ankle or spine that is responsible for the patient's pain may yield disastrous results. The major complication of intra-articular injection of the midtarsal joints is infection. This complication should be exceedingly rare if strict aseptic technique is adhered to. Approximately 25% of patients will complain of a transient increase in pain after intra-articular injection of the midtarsal joints and should be warned of such.

CLINICAL PEARLS

Pain emanating from the midtarsal joints is commonly seen in football punters and ballet dancers, both of whom forcefully point their toes. This injection technique is extremely effective in the treatment of pain secondary to the causes of arthritis of the midtarsal joint mentioned. Coexistent bursitis and tendinitis may also contribute to midtarsal joint pain and may require additional treatment with more localized injection of a local anesthetic and depot-steroid. This technique is a safe procedure if careful attention is paid to the clinically relevant anatomy in the areas to be injected. Care must be taken to use sterile technique to avoid infection, as well as the use of universal precautions to avoid risk to the operator. The incidence of ecchymosis and hematoma formation can be decreased if pressure is placed on the injection site immediately after injection. The use of physical modalities, including local heat as well as gentle range of motion exercises, should be introduced several days after the patient undergoes this injection technique for midtarsal pain. Vigorous exercises should be avoided because they will exacerbate the patient's symptomatology. Simple analgesics and nonsteroidal anti-inflammatory agents may be used concurrently with this injection technique.

66 Achilles Bursitis

ICD-9 CODE 727.00

THE CLINICAL SYNDROME

Achilles bursitis is being seen with increasing frequency in clinical practice as jogging has increased in popularity. The Achilles tendon is susceptible to the development of bursitis both at its insertion on the calcaneus and at its narrowest part at a point approximately 5 cm above its insertion. Additionally, the Achilles tendon is subject to repetitive motion injury that may result in microtrauma, which heals poorly due to the tendon's avascular nature. Running is often implicated as the inciting factor of acute Achilles bursitis. Bursitis of the Achilles tendon frequently coexists with Achilles tendinitis, creating additional pain and functional disability. Calcium deposition around the Achilles bursa may occur if the inflammation continues, making subsequent treatment more difficult.

SIGNS AND SYMPTOMS

The onset of Achilles bursitis is usually acute, occurring after overuse or misuse of the ankle joint. Inciting factors may include activities such as running, sudden stopping, and starting as when playing tennis (Fig. 66–1). Improper stretching of the gastrocnemius and Achilles tendons before exercise has also been implicated in the development of Achilles bursitis as well as acute tendinitis and tendon rupture. The pain of Achilles bursitis is constant and severe and is localized in the posterior ankle. Significant sleep disturbance is often reported. The patient may attempt to splint the inflamed Achilles bursa by adopting a flat-footed gait to avoid plantarflexion of the affected foot. Patients with Achilles bursitis will exhibit pain with resisted plan-

tarflexion of the foot. A creaking or grating sensation may be palpated when passively plantarflexing the foot due to coexistent tendinitis. As mentioned, the chronically inflamed Achilles tendon may suddenly rupture with stress or during vigorous injection procedures to treat Achilles bursitis.

TESTING

Plain radiographs are indicated in all patients who present with posterior ankle pain. Based on the patient's clinical presentation, additional testing including complete blood cell count, sedimentation rate, and antinuclear antibody testing may be indicated. Magnetic resonance imaging (MRI) of the ankle is indicated if joint instability is suspected. Radionucleotide bone scanning is useful to identify stress fractures of the tibia not seen on plain radiographs. The following injection technique serves as both a diagnostic and therapeutic maneuver.

DIFFERENTIAL DIAGNOSIS

Achilles bursitis is generally easily identified on clinical grounds. Because tendinitis frequently accompanies Achilles bursitis, the specific diagnosis may be unclear. Stress fractures of the ankle may also mimic Achilles bursitis and tendinitis and may be identified on plain radiographs, MRI, or radionucleotide bone scanning.

TREATMENT

Initial treatment of the pain and functional disability associated with Achilles bursitis should include a combination of the nonsteroidal anti-inflammatory agents or cyclooxygenase-2 (COX-2) inhibitors and physical therapy. The local application of heat and cold may also be beneficial. Avoidance of repetitive activities responsible for the evolution of the bursitis, such as jogging, should be encouraged. For patients

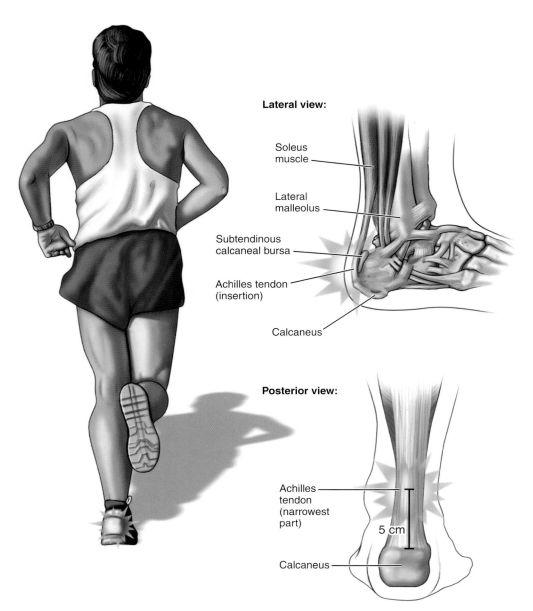

Lateral view:

Soleus muscle

Lateral malleolus

Subtendinous calcaneal bursa

Achilles tendon (insertion)

Calcaneus

Posterior view:

Achilles tendon (narrowest part)

5 cm

Calcaneus

Figure 66–1

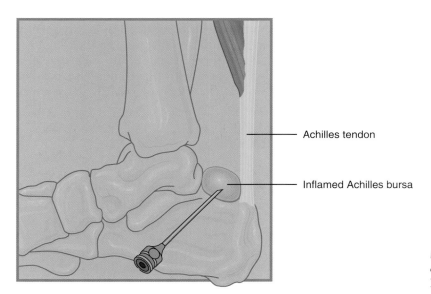

Achilles tendon

Inflamed Achilles bursa

Figure 66–2. (From Waldman SD: Atlas of Pain Management Injection Techniques. Philadelphia, WB Saunders, 2000, p 329.)

who do not respond to these treatment modalities, the following injection technique with a local anesthetic and steroid may be a reasonable next step.

Injection for Achilles bursitis is carried out by placing the patient in the prone position with the affected foot hanging off the end of the table. The foot is gently dorsiflexed to facilitate identification of the margin of the tendon to aid in avoiding injection directly into the tendon. The tender points at the tendinous insertion and/or at its narrowest part approximately 5 cm above the insertion are identified and marked with a sterile marker.

Proper preparation with antiseptic solution of the skin overlying these points is then carried out. A sterile syringe containing 2.0 mL of 0.25% preservative-free bupivacaine and 40 mg of methylprednisolone is attached to a 25-gauge $1\frac{1}{2}$-inch needle using strict aseptic technique. With strict aseptic technique, the previously marked points are palpated. The needle is then carefully advanced at this point alongside the tendon through the skin and subcutaneous tissues with care being taken not to enter the substance of the tendon (Fig. 66–2). The contents of the syringe are then gently injected while slowly withdrawing the needle. There should be minimal resistance to injection. If there is significant resistance to injection, the needle tip is probably in the substance of the Achilles tendon and should be withdrawn slightly until the injection proceeds without significant resistance. The needle is then removed, and a sterile pressure dressing and ice pack are placed at the injection site.

COMPLICATIONS AND PITFALLS

The possibility of trauma to the Achilles tendon from the injection itself remains an ever-present possibility. Tendons that are highly inflamed or previously damaged are subject to rupture if they are directly injected. This complication can be greatly decreased if the clinician uses gentle technique and stops injecting immediately if significant resistance to injection is encountered. Approximately 25% of patients will complain of a transient increase in pain after this injection technique and should be warned of such.

CLINICAL PEARLS

The Achilles tendon is the thickest and strongest tendon in the body, yet it also is very susceptible to rupture. The common tendon of the gastrocnemius muscle, the Achilles tendon begins at midcalf and continues downward to attach to the posterior calcaneus, where it may become inflamed. The Achilles tendon narrows during this downward course, becoming most narrow approximately 5 cm above its calcaneal insertion. It is at this narrowmost point that tendinitis and bursitis may also occur. The above-mentioned injection technique is extremely effective in the treatment of pain secondary to the above-mentioned causes of posterior ankle pain. Coexistent tendinitis and arthritis may also contribute to posterior ankle pain and may require additional treatment with a more localized injection of a local anesthetic and depot-steroid.

The technique is a safe procedure if careful attention is paid to the clinically relevant anatomy in the areas to be injected. The use of physical modalities, including local heat as well as gentle range of motion exercises, should be introduced several days after the patient undergoes this injection technique for ankle pain. Vigorous exercises should be avoided because they will exacerbate the patient's symptomatology. Simple analgesics and nonsteroidal anti-inflammatory agents may be used concurrently with this injection technique.

67 Talofibular Pain Syndrome

ICD-9 CODE 845.09

THE CLINICAL SYNDROME

Talofibular pain syndrome is being encountered more frequently in clinical practice with the increased interest in jogging and marathon running. The talofibular ligament is susceptible to strain from acute injury from sudden inversion of the ankle or from repetitive microtrauma to the ligament from overuse or misuse such as long distance running on soft or uneven surfaces (Fig. 67–1). Patients with strain of the talofibular ligament will complain of pain just below the lateral malleolus. Activities that require inversion of the ankle joint will exacerbate the pain.

SIGNS AND SYMPTOMS

On physical examination, there will be point tenderness just below the lateral malleolus. With acute trauma, ecchymosis over the ligament may be noted. Passive inversion of the ankle joint will exacerbate the pain. Coexistent bursitis and arthritis of the ankle and subtalar joint may also be present and confuse the clinical picture. Stress fractures of the foot also occur with increased frequency in runners, and this must be considered in all patients thought to have talofibular pain syndrome.

TESTING

Plain radiographs are indicated in all patients who present with ankle pain. Based on the patient's clinical presentation, additional testing including complete blood cell count, sedimentation rate, and antinuclear antibody testing may be indicated. Magnetic resonance imaging (MRI) of the ankle is indicated if disruption of the talofibular ligament or joint instability, occult mass, or tumor is suspected.

DIFFERENTIAL DIAGNOSIS

Avulsion fractures of the calcaneus, talus, lateral malleolus, and the base of the fifth metatarsal can mimic the pain of injury to the talofibular ligament. Bursitis and tendinitis as well as gout of the midtarsal joints may coexist with ligament strain and may confuse the diagnosis. Tarsal tunnel syndrome may occur after ankle trauma and may further confuse the clinical picture.

TREATMENT

Initial treatment of the pain and functional disability associated with talofibular pain syndrome should include a combination of the nonsteroidal anti-inflammatory agents or cyclooxygenase-2 (COX-2) inhibitors and physical therapy. The local application of heat and cold may also be beneficial. Avoidance of repetitive activities that aggravate the patient's symptomatology as well as short-term immobilization of the ankle joint may also provide relief. For patients who do not respond to these treatment modalities, the injection of the talofibular ligament may be a reasonable next step.

COMPLICATIONS AND PITFALLS

Failure to identify occult fractures of the ankle and foot may result in significant morbidity. Radionucleotide bone scanning and MRI of the ankle should be performed on all patients experiencing unexplained ankle and foot pain, especially if trauma is present. The major complication of the above injection technique is infection. This complication should be exceedingly rare if strict aseptic technique is adhered to. Approximately 25% of patients will

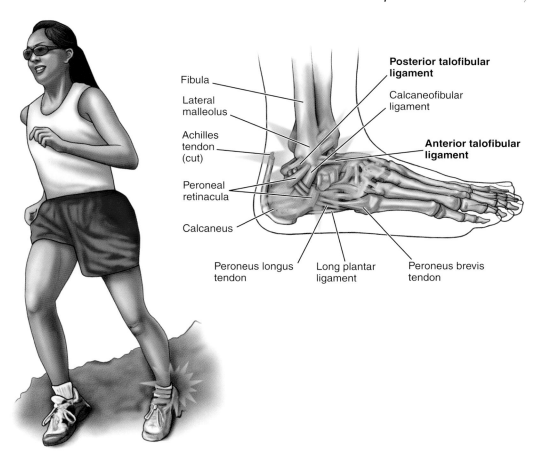

Fibula

Lateral
malleolus

Achilles
tendon
(cut)

Peroneal
retinacula

Calcaneus

**Posterior talofibular
ligament**

Calcaneofibular
ligament

**Anterior talofibular
ligament**

Peroneus longus
tendon

Long plantar
ligament

Peroneus brevis
tendon

Figure 67–1

complain of a transient increase in pain after injection of the talofibular ligament and should be warned of such. Injection around strained ligaments should always be done gently to avoid further damage to the already compromised ligament.

CLINICAL PEARLS

It is estimated that approximately 25,000 people sprain their ankles every day. Although viewed as benign by the lay public, ankle sprains can result in significant permanent pain and disability. The major ligaments of the ankle joint include the deltoid, anterior talofibular, calcaneofibular, and posterior talofibular ligaments, which provide the majority of strength to the ankle joint. The talofibular ligament is not as strong as the deltoid ligament and is suscep-tible to strain. The talofibular ligament runs from the anterior border of the lateral malleolus to the lateral surface of the talus.

The injection technique mentioned is extremely effective in the treatment of pain secondary to the talofibular ligament strain. Coexistent arthritis, bursitis, and tendinitis may also contribute to medial ankle pain and may require additional treatment with more localized injection of a local anesthetic and depot-steroid. The use of physical modalities, including local heat as well as gentle range of motion exercises, should be introduced several days after the patient undergoes this injection technique for ankle pain. Vigorous exercises should be avoided because they will exacerbate the patient's symptomatology. Simple analgesics and nonsteroidal anti-inflammatory agents may be used concurrently with this injection technique.

68 *Fibulocalcaneal Pain Syndrome*

ICD-9 CODE 845.09

THE CLINICAL SYNDROME

Fibulocalcaneal pain syndrome is the result of injury to the fibulocalcaneal ligament, usually due to sudden inversion of the ankle as when stepping off a high curb (Fig. 68–1). The fibulocalcaneal ligament is also susceptible to strain from acute injury from repetitive microtrauma to the ligament from overuse or misuse such as long distance running on soft or uneven surfaces. Patients with fibulocalcaneal pain syndrome will complain of pain anterior and inferior to the lateral malleolus. Inversion of the ankle joint will exacerbate the pain.

SIGNS AND SYMPTOMS

On physical examination, there will be point tenderness just below the lateral malleolus. With acute trauma, ecchymosis over the ligament may be noted. Passive inversion of the ankle joint will exacerbate the pain. Coexistent bursitis and arthritis of the ankle and subtalar joint may also be present and confuse the clinical picture. Stress fractures of the foot also occur with increased frequency in runners, and this must be considered in all patients thought to have fibulocalcaneal pain syndrome.

TESTING

Plain radiographs are indicated in all patients who present with ankle pain. Based on the patient's clinical presentation, additional testing including complete blood cell count, sedimentation rate, and antinuclear antibody testing may be indicated. Magnetic resonance imaging (MRI) of the ankle is indi-cated if disruption of the fibulocalcaneal ligament or joint instability, occult mass, or tumor is suspected.

DIFFERENTIAL DIAGNOSIS

Avulsion fractures of the calcaneus, talus, lateral malleolus, and the base of the fifth metatarsal can mimic the pain of injury to the fibulocalcaneal ligament. Bursitis and tendinitis as well as gout of the midtarsal joints may coexist with ligament strain and may con-fuse the diagnosis. Tarsal tunnel syndrome may occur after ankle trauma and may further confuse the clinical picture.

TREATMENT

Initial treatment of the pain and functional disability associated with fibulocalcaneal pain syndrome should include a combination of the nonsteroidal anti-inflammatory agents or cyclooxygenase-2 (COX-2) inhibitors and physical therapy. The local application of heat and cold may also be beneficial. Avoidance of repetitive activities that aggravate the patient's symptomatology as well as short-term immobilization of the ankle joint may also provide relief. For patients who do not respond to these treatment modalities, the injection of the fibulocalcaneal ligament may be a reasonable next step.

COMPLICATIONS AND PITFALLS

Failure to identify occult fractures of the ankle and foot may result in significant morbidity. Radio-nucleotide bone scanning and MRI of the ankle should be performed on all patients experiencing unexplained ankle and foot pain, especially if trauma is present. The major complication of the above injection technique is infection. This complication should be exceedingly rare if strict aseptic technique is adhered to. Approximately 25% of patients will

245

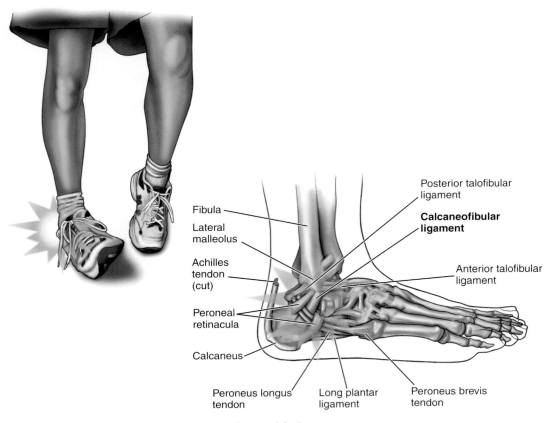

Figure 68–1

complain of a transient increase in pain after injection of the fibulocalcaneal ligament and should be warned of such. Injection around strained ligaments should always be done gently to avoid further damage to the already compromised ligament.

CLINICAL PEARLS

It is estimated that approximately 25,000 people sprain their ankles every day. Although viewed as benign by the lay public, ankle sprains can result in significant permanent pain and disability. The major ligaments of the ankle joint include the deltoid, anterior talofibular, calcaneofibular, and posterior talofibular ligaments, which provide the majority of strength to the ankle joint.

Injection of the fibulocalcaneal ligament is extremely effective in the treatment of pain secondary to the fibulocalcaneal ligament strain. Coexistent arthritis, bursitis, and tendinitis may also contribute to medial ankle pain and may require additional treatment with more localized injection of a local anesthetic and depot-steroid. The use of physical modalities, including local heat as well as gentle range of motion exercises, should be introduced several days after the patient undergoes this injection technique for ankle pain. Vigorous exercises should be avoided because they will exacerbate the patient's symptomatology. Simple analgesics and nonsteroidal anti-inflammatory agents may be used concurrently with this injection technique.

69 *Bunionette Pain*

ICD-9 CODE 727.1

THE CLINICAL SYNDROME

Occurring less commonly than the common bunion, bunionette is a common cause of lateral foot pain. The term *bunionette* refers to a constellation of symptoms including soft tissue swelling over the fifth metatarsophalangeal joint associated with abnormal angulation of the joint resulting in a prominent fifth metatarsal head with associated medial angulation. Bunionette is also known as *Tailor's bunion.* This deformity is analogous to the hallux valgus deformity and also occurs more commonly in females. The development of an inflamed adventitious bursa may accompany bunionette formation and contribute to the patient's pain. A corn overlying the fifth metatarsal head is also usually present. The most common cause of bunionette formation is the wearing of tight narrow-toed shoes (Fig. 69–1). High heels may exacerbate the problem.

SIGNS AND SYMPTOMS

The majority of patients presenting with bunionette will present with the complaint of pain that is localized to the affected fifth metatarsophalangeal joint and the inability to get shoes to fit. Walking makes the pain worse, with rest and heat providing some relief. The pain is constant and characterized as aching in nature. The pain may interfere with sleep. Some patients will complain of a grating or popping sensation with use of the joint, and crepitus may be present on physical examination. Physical examination will reveal soft tissue swelling over the fifth metatarsophalangeal joint associated with abnormal angulation of the joint resulting in a prominent fifth metatarsal head with associated medial angulation.

TESTING

Plain radiographs are indicated in all patients who present with bunionette pain. Based on the patient's clinical presentation, additional testing including complete blood cell count, sedimentation rate, and antinuclear antibody testing may be indicated. Magnetic resonance imaging (MRI) of the fifth metatarsophalangeal joint is indicated if joint instability, occult mass, or tumor is suspected.

DIFFERENTIAL DIAGNOSIS

The diagnosis of bunionette is usually obvious on clinical grounds alone. Complicating the care of the patient suffering from a typical bunion deformity is the fact that bursitis and tendinitis of the foot and ankle frequently coexist with the bunion pain. Furthermore, stress fractures of the metatarsals, phalanges, and/or sesamoid bones may also confuse the clinical diagnosis and require specific treatment.

TESTING

Plain radiographs are indicated in all patients who present with bunionette pain. Based on the patient's clinical presentation, additional testing including complete blood cell count, sedimentation rate, and antinuclear antibody testing may be indicated. Magnetic resonance imaging (MRI) of the toe is indicated if joint instability, occult mass, or tumor is suspected.

TREATMENT

Initial treatment of the pain and functional disability associated with bunionette deformity should include a combination of the nonsteroidal anti-inflammatory agents or cyclooxygenase-2 (COX-2) inhibitors and physical therapy. The local application of heat and cold may also be beneficial. Avoidance

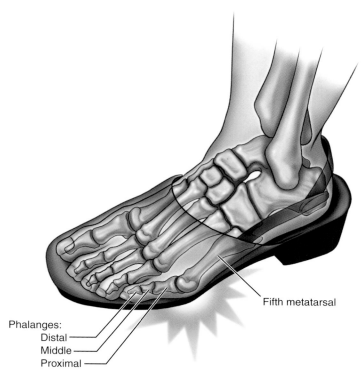

Phalanges:
    Distal
    Middle
    Proximal

Fifth metatarsal

Figure 69–1

of repetitive activities that aggravate the patient's symptomatology as well as avoidance of narrow-toed or high-heeled shoes combined with short-term immobilization of the affected toes may also provide relief. For patients who do not respond to these treatment modalities, an injection with a local anesthetic and steroid may be a reasonable next step.

SIDE EFFECTS AND PITFALLS

Failure to identify primary or metastatic tumor of the foot that is responsible for the patient's pain may yield disastrous results. The major complication of the above injection technique is infection. This complication should be exceedingly rare if strict aseptic technique is adhered to. Approximately 25% of patients will complain of a transient increase in pain after this technique and should be warned of such.

CLINICAL PEARLS

Pain from bunionette can be quite debilitating and the deformity cosmetically unacceptable for many patients. Injection of the bunionette with a local anesthetic and steroid is extremely effective in the treatment of pain secondary to bunionette. Coexistent arthritis, bursitis, and tendinitis may also contribute to bunionette pain and may require additional treatment with more localized injection of a local anesthetic and depot-steroid.

Patients with bunionette should be advised to avoid tight, narrow-toed shoes. The use of physical modalities, including local heat as well as gentle range of motion exercises, should be introduced several days after the patient undergoes this injection technique for toe pain. Vigorous exercises should be avoided because they will exacerbate the patient's symptomatology. Simple analgesics and nonsteroidal anti-inflammatory agents may be used concurrently with this injection technique.

70 *Sesamoiditis*

ICD-9 CODE 733.99

THE CLINICAL SYNDROME

Sesamoiditis is being seen with increasing frequency in clinical practice owing to the increased interest in jogging and long distance running. The sesamoid bones are small, rounded structures that are embedded in the flexor tendons of the foot and are usually in close proximity to the joints. These sesamoid bones serve to decrease friction and pressure of the flexor tendon as it passes in proximity to a joint. Sesamoid bones of the first metatarsal occur in almost all patients, with sesamoid bones being present in the flexor tendons of the second and fifth metatarsals in a significant number of patients.

Although the sesamoid bone associated with the first metatarsal head is affected most commonly, the sesamoid bones of the second and fifth metatarsal heads are also subject to the development of sesamoiditis. Sesamoiditis is characterized by tenderness and pain over the metatarsal heads. The patient often feels that they are walking with a stone in their shoe (Fig. 70–1). The pain of sesamoiditis worsens with prolonged standing or walking for long distances and is exacerbated by improperly fitting or padded shoes. Sesamoiditis is most often associated with pushing-off injuries during football or repetitive microtrauma from running or dancing.

SIGNS AND SYMPTOMS

On physical examination, pain can be reproduced by pressure on the affected sesamoid bone. In contradistinction to metatarsalgia, where the tender area remains over the metatarsal heads, with sesamoiditis, the area of maximum tenderness will move along with the flexor tendon when the patient actively flexes his or her toe. The patient with sesamoiditis will often exhibit an antalgic gait in an effort to

reduce weight bearing during walking. With acute trauma to the sesamoid, ecchymosis over the plantar surface of the foot may be present.

TESTING

Plain radiographs are indicated in all patients who present with sesamoiditis to rule out fractures and to identify sesamoid bones that may have become inflamed. Based on the patient's clinical presentation, additional testing including complete blood cell count, sedimentation rate, and antinuclear antibody testing may be indicated. Magnetic resonance imaging (MRI) of the metatarsal bones is indicated if joint instability, occult mass, or tumor is suspected. Radionucleotide bone scanning may be useful in identifying stress fractures of the metatarsal bones or sesamoid bones that may be missed on plain radiographs of the foot.

DIFFERENTIAL DIAGNOSIS

Primary pathology of the foot, including gout and occult fractures, may mimic the pain and disability associated with sesamoiditis. Entrapment neuropathies such as tarsal tunnel syndrome may also confuse the diagnosis, as may bursitis and plantar fasciitis of the foot, both of which may coexist with sesamoiditis. Metatarsalgia is another common cause of forefoot pain and may be distinguished from sesamoiditis by the fact that the pain of metatarsalgia is over the metatarsal heads and does not move when the patient actively flexes his or her toes as is the case with sesamoiditis. Primary and metastatic tumors of the foot may also present in a manner analogous to arthritis of the midtarsal joints.

TREATMENT

Initial treatment of the pain and functional disability associated with sesamoiditis should include a

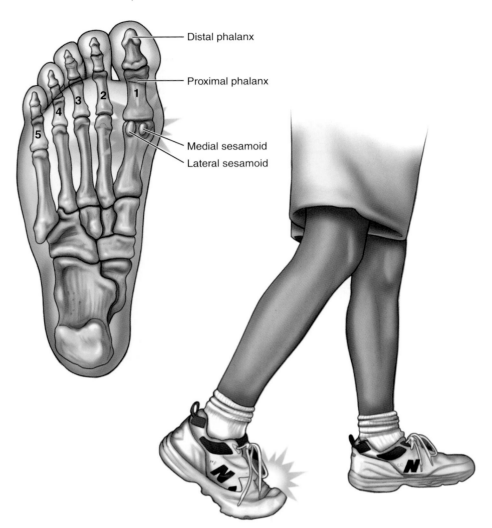

Distal phalanx

Proximal phalanx

Medial sesamoid
Lateral sesamoid

Figure 70–1

combination of the nonsteroidal anti-inflammatory agents or cyclooxygenase-2 (COX-2) inhibitors and physical therapy. The local application of heat and cold may also be beneficial. Avoidance of repetitive activities that aggravate the patient's symptomatology as well as short-term immobilization of the midtarsal joint may also provide relief. For patients who do not respond to these treatment modalities, injection of the affected sesamoid bone with a local anesthetic and steroid may be a reasonable next step.

SIDE EFFECTS AND PITFALLS

The major complication of injection of sesamoiditis is infection. This complication should be exceedingly rare if strict aseptic technique is adhered to. Approximately 25% of patients will complain of a transient increase in pain after injection of sesamoid bones and should be warned of such. Another potential risk of this injection technique is trauma to the tendon from the injection itself.

CLINICAL PEARLS

Pain emanating from the forefoot is a common problem encountered in clinical practice. Sesamoidi-

tis must be distinguished from stress fractures of the metatarsal bones, metatarsalgia, Morton's neuroma, and fractures of the sesamoid bones. Although the injection technique mentioned will provide palliation of the pain of sesamoiditis, the patient will often also require shoe orthoses that include padded insoles to help remove pressure from the affected sesamoid bones. Coexistent bursitis and tendinitis may also contribute to metatarsal pain and may require additional treatment with more localized injection of an anesthetic and depot-steroid. The use of physical modalities, including local heat as well as gentle range of motion exercises, should be introduced several days after the patient undergoes this injection technique for sesamoiditis pain. Vigorous exercises should be avoided because they will exacerbate the patient's symptomatology. Simple analgesics and nonsteroidal anti-inflammatory agents may be used concurrently with this injection technique.

71 *Metatarsalgia*

THE CLINICAL SYNDROME

Along with sesamoiditis, metatarsalgia is another painful condition of the forefoot that is being seen with increasing frequency in clinical practice owing to the increased interest in jogging and long distance running. Metatarsalgia is characterized by tenderness and pain over the metatarsal heads. Patients often feel that they are walking with a stone in their shoe. The pain of metatarsalgia worsens with prolonged standing or walking for long distances and is exacerbated by improperly fitting or padded shoes. Often the patient suffering from metatarsalgia will develop hard callus formation over the heads of the second and third metatarsal as they try to shift the weight off the head of the first metatarsal to relieve the pain. This callus formation increases the pressure on the metatarsal heads and further exacerbates the patient's pain and disability.

SIGNS AND SYMPTOMS

On physical examination, pain can be reproduced by pressure on the metatarsal heads (Fig. 71–1). Callus formation will often be present over the heads of the second and third metatarsal heads and can be distinguished from plantar warts by the lack of thrombosed blood vessels that appear as small dark spots through the substance of the wart when the surface is trimmed. The patient with metatarsalgia will often exhibit an antalgic gait in an effort to reduce weight bearing during the static stance phase of walking. Ligamentous laxity and flattening of the transverse arch may also be present, giving the foot a splayed-out appearance.

TESTING

Plain radiographs are indicated in all patients who present with metatarsalgia to rule out fractures and to identify sesamoid bones that may have become inflamed. Based on the patient's clinical presentation, additional testing including complete blood cell count, sedimentation rate, and antinuclear antibody testing may be indicated. Magnetic resonance imaging (MRI) of the metatarsal bones is indicated if joint instability, occult mass, or tumor is suspected. Radionucleotide bone scanning may be useful in identifying stress fractures that may be missed on plain radiographs of the foot.

DIFFERENTIAL DIAGNOSIS

Primary pathology of the foot, including gout and occult fractures, may mimic the pain and disability associated with metatarsalgia (Fig. 71–2). Entrapment neuropathies such as tarsal tunnel syndrome may also confuse the diagnosis, as may bursitis and plantar fasciitis of the foot, both of which may coexist with sesamoiditis. Sesamoid bones beneath the heads of the metatarsal bones are present in some individuals and are subject to the development of inflammation called *sesamoiditis*. Sesamoiditis is another common cause of forefoot pain and may be distinguished from metatarsalgia by the fact that the pain of metatarsalgia is centered over the patient's metatarsal heads and does not move when the patient actively flexes his or her toes as is the case with sesamoiditis. The muscles of the metatarsal joints and their attaching tendons are also susceptible to trauma and to wear and tear from overuse and misuse and may contribute to forefoot pain. Primary and metastatic tumors of the foot may also present in a manner analogous to arthritis of the midtarsal joints.

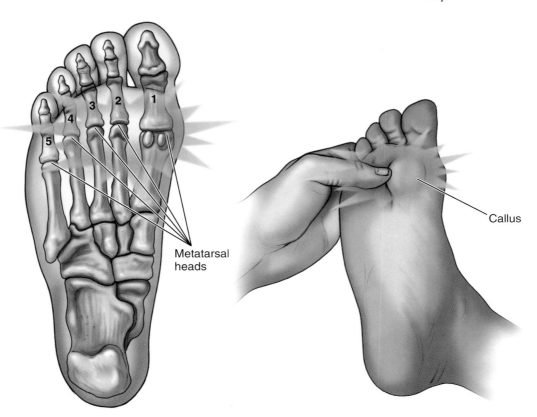

Metatarsal
heads

Callus

Figure 71–1

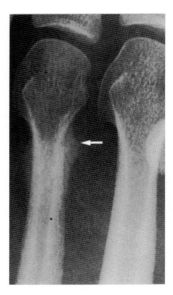

Figure 71–2. Stress fracture of the metatarsal ("march fracture"). Anteroposterior radiograph demonstrates fluffy periosteal new bone along the distal shaft of the third metatarsal (*arrow*); the patient had foot pain for 16 days. (From Grainger RG, Allison D: Grainger & Allison's Diagnostic Radiology: A Textbook of Medical Imaging, 3rd ed. New York, Churchill Livingstone, 1997, p 1610.)

TREATMENT

Initial treatment of the pain and functional disability associated with metatarsalgia should include a combination of the nonsteroidal anti-inflammatory agents or cyclooxygenase-2 (COX-2) inhibitors and physical therapy. The local application of heat and cold may also be beneficial. Avoidance of repetitive activities that aggravate the patient's symptomatology as well as short-term immobilization of the midtarsal joint may also provide relief. For patients who do not respond to these treatment modalities, injection of the affected metatarsal heads with a local anesthetic and steroid may be a reasonable next step.

SIDE EFFECTS AND PITFALLS

The major complication of injection of the metatarsal heads is infection. This complication should be exceedingly rare if strict aseptic technique is adhered to. Approximately 25% of patients will complain of a transient increase in pain after injection of the metatarsal heads and should be warned of such. Another potential risk of this injection technique is trauma to the associated tendons from the injection itself.

CLINICAL PEARLS

Pain emanating from the forefoot is a common problem encountered in clinical practice. Metatarsalgia must be distinguished from stress fractures of the metatarsal bones, Morton's neuroma, and sesamoiditis. Although the injection technique mentioned will provide palliation of the pain of metatarsalgia, the patient will often also require shoe orthoses, including metatarsal bars and padded insoles, to help remove pressure from the metatarsal heads. Coexistent bursitis and tendinitis may also contribute to metatarsal pain and may require additional treatment with more localized injection of a local anesthetic and depot-steroid. Injection of the metatarsal heads with a local anesthetic and steroid is a safe procedure if careful attention is paid to the clinically relevant anatomy in the areas to be injected. The use of physical modalities, including local heat as well as gentle range of motion exercises, should be introduced several days after the patient undergoes this injection technique for metatarsalgia pain. Vigorous exercises should be avoided because they will exacerbate the patient's symptomatology. Simple analgesics and nonsteroidal anti-inflammatory agents may be used concurrently with this injection technique.

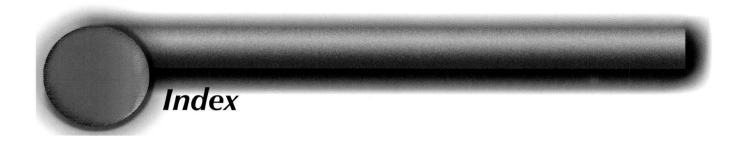

Index

Note: Page numbers followed by the letter f refer to figures.